OUTCOMES INTO
CLINICAL PRACTICE

OUTCOMES INTO CLINICAL PRACTICE

Edited by Tony Delamothe

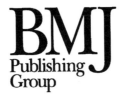

BMJ Publishing Group

First published in 1994
Reprinted 1995
by the BMJ Publishing Group, BMA House, Tavistock Square,
London WC1H 9JR

British Library Cataloguing in Publication Data

A catalogue record for this book is available
from the British Library

ISBN 0-7279-0888-X

Typeset in Great Britain by Apek Typesetters Ltd., Nailsea, Bristol
Printed and bound in Great Britain by Latimer Trend & Company Ltd, Plymouth

Contents

Preface

Doctors have always been interested in the results of what they do. So what explains the burgeoning "clinical outcomes" industry, with its own gurus, guides, and gatherings?

This book emerged from one such gathering (organised by the BMA, the BMJ Publishing Group, and the UK Clearing House for Information on the Assessment of Health Outcomes). What is obvious from almost every chapter is that doctors' interest in the outcomes of their care has been a pretty haphazard affair. Systematic evaluation of practice (outside clinical trials) has been rare; evaluation from the perspective of patients has been even rarer. *Outcomes into Clinical Practice* highlights what we have been missing.

As its title suggests, the point of the book (and the conference on which it was based) was not to provide yet another critical commentary on medical care but to consider how the results of outcomes research could be fed back into clinical practice. Taking us beyond theory are case studies – from medicine, surgery, general practice, community services, and mental health – showing the technique in action.

Many of those involved with these projects would readily admit that they have taken only the first tentative steps towards collecting and using data on outcomes. Fortunately, the official climate in Britain is very supportive of such activity. Enthusiastically endorsing outcomes research in his introductory chapter, England's chief medical officer, Kenneth Calman, lists more than two pages of Department of Health initiatives related to outcomes (many began during his tenure). Together, these initiatives have stimulated "a more self questioning culture."

In the next chapter Albert Mulley from Massachusetts General Hospital expands on the potential of outcomes research and shows how it might be applied to benign prostatic hyperplasia. The basic premise of outcomes research is that when recommending treatment doctors need to know what are the likely outcomes of different treatments and what matters to individual patients. Only systematic research can provide this information, and patient preference is crucial. For example, in Mulley's example patients with benign prostatic hyperplasia may value identical outcomes differently, assigning very different relative values to urinary dysfunction (or its relief) and to sexual function (or its compromise). Unless clinical decisions consider patients' preferences "we run the risk of providing treatment to patients who do not value the expected outcome while withholding it from those who do," said Mulley. In other words, one man not much bothered by his symptoms might end up with major surgery (and its attendant risks); another, greatly bothered by symptoms, might be refused surgery.

There are other advantages of outcomes research in addition to those that help doctors and patients decide about individual treatment. Data on how people value alternative outcomes can inform policy decisions such as the allocation of resources. Outcomes can be compared between providers and used to identify best practice and to develop practice guidelines. Such data can be used to distinguish appropriate and desirable variations in practice from those that are neither. And lastly, and perhaps most importantly, rigorous comparisons of outcomes across providers and processes of care allow the medical profession to update continuously its knowledge base, thereby providing a scientific basis for professional self assessment and improvement.

It was variations in the management of benign prostatic disease (and variations in the outcomes of such management) that convinced researchers that here was a problem worthy of further study. In a later chapter, Klim McPherson, of the London School of Hygiene and Tropical Medicine, returns to the role of the prostate in outcomes research. (Perhaps future medical students will include "precipitating outcomes research" among the prostate's otherwise murky functions in answers to exam questions.)

Several themes recur in subsequent chapters - most notably

which data to collect and how to interpret them. Marianne Rigge of the College of Health points out the attraction of collecting the options that are easiest to measure, such as uncomplicated recovery from surgery. Yet outcomes measured in trials may not be those of most concern to patients. Mark Williams from the University of Bristol concurs: "outcome assessment has been hampered by a lack of standardised terminology, missing or non-quantifiable clinical information, small samples, short periods of follow up, and emphasis on physicians' definitions of relief of pain and on measures of technical success rather than on patients' satisfaction or quality of life." To prove his point he lists the components of 15 scales that grade the results of total hip replacement: global assessment (from the patient's point of view) is missing from all but one of them.

Writing of patients with asthma Nottinghamshire general practitioner Mike Pringle regrets that no easy standardised tools are available to measure quality of life, activity levels, social functioning, psychological distress, patients' perception of their asthma, and objective symptom control – "but most practitioners rate them highly as quality markers." He describes his practice's approach to assessing outcomes: each month it discusses "significant events" – that is, every stroke, myocardial infarction, new diagnosis of cancer, suicide attempt, unplanned pregnancy, patient leaving the practice without changing address, visit accepted but not done, patient waiting over 30 minutes after the appointment time – and so on. "They are all outcomes of the clinical and administrative commitment of the practice. We look at each of these events and ask was everything possible done that should have been done?"

The book suggests that outcome measures may be proliferating out of control; but is that good or bad? Without trying different approaches to outcome assessment we will not be able to assess the best ways forward, believe Martin Bardsley and Robert Cleary, based on their experience of assessing knee replacements at Newcastle's Freeman Hospital. "We may be better advised to have less comparability between sites at least until we find out what works best."

But what James Raftery of the University of Southampton says of the limitations of data on cost effectiveness also seems relevant to outcome measures generally. Each evaluation of cost effectiveness tends to start from scratch rather than be built on shared approaches, which might be applied routinely and cheaply, he says. "We need more development, less research."

These are still very early days for outcomes research – in Britain or anywhere – and at this stage the benefits of diversity probably outweigh the disadvantages. It's easy to forget how recently the subject has attracted attention: for the first 40 years of its existence the NHS had no explicitly defined outcomes (an anomaly corrected only by the publication of *Health of the Nation*).

The contributors to this volume are shining their lights in many different directions. And in a decade's time it's unlikely that outcomes research will bear much resemblance to what they help us to glimpse today. Nevertheless, even these glimpses are grounds for excitement. As Mulley argues in his chapter, few conditions would not be better treated if we developed a system of outcomes research that could be brought into clinical practice.

TONY DELAMOTHE

1 Introduction

KENNETH CALMAN

In introducing this topic I hope to discuss its importance; provide an overview of the key clinical questions and issues concerning outcomes; and describe some of the Department of Health's own contributions to addressing these issues. The issues are covered in much more detail in the papers that follow. I am going to illustrate the key questions and issues using two examples – diabetes and cancer. At the outset it is important to note that the purpose of clinical outcomes is to improve the health and health care of the population.

I find the wording of the topic slightly odd, particularly the word "into." Surely outcomes are part of clinical practice. Outcomes assessment has been part of good clinical practice for

---

Sick children 'are getting raw deal in NHS hospitals'

Children account for one in seven hospital admissions and about £1.4bn, or 10 per cent of spending on hospital and community health services. But the outcomes of treatments on children are not routinely monitored. Despite a consensus among medical researchers on the need to treat children at home where feasible, some hospital procedures carried out on them are of doubtful value, the Audit Commission said.

Glue ear, one of the most common childhood complaints, is generally treated surgically by adenoidectomy or a myringotomy (incision of the eardrum). But several studies have found that up to one-third of these operations are carried out unnecessarily because of spontaneous natural recovery....

The Independent 3 February 1993

---

centuries. Most clinical professionals think about the benefit they offer to patients and undertake some follow up to check results as an essential part of clinical practice.

So why is there this renewed concern about outcomes? The newspaper headline in the box and the story's contents are typical of many that we see regularly.

It raises questions and concerns about the resources going into child health care, about outcomes of this resource use, and about value for money.

Such public concern should also be a concern for clinical professionals. The professions have as much a vested interest in ensuring that the clinical care provided is of the highest possible standard and quality. A key challenge is demonstrating such achievement with data on outcomes and using outcomes data to shape and improve quality.

Key clinical questions and issues

Table 1.1 shows data on mortality due to diabetes, standardised for age and sex, by regional health authority in England. There is considerable variation in mortality which is considered potentially

Table 1.1 Standardised mortality ratios for diabetes in male patients aged 1–44 years, 1988–92

	No. observed	Standardised mortality ratio (95% confidence interval)	
England and Wales	441	100	
England	423	101	(92 to 112)
Regional health authority:			
Northern	34	128	(89 to 179)
Yorkshire	32	101	(69 to 143)
Trent	32	78	(53 to 110)
East Anglian	16	91	(52 to 147)
North West Thames	28	87	(58 to 126)
North East Thames	32	97	(66 to 136)
South East Thames	28	89	(59 to 128)
South West Thames	17	64	(37 to 103)
Wessex	23	91	(58 to 137)
Oxford	23	98	(62 to 147)
South Western	30	110	(74 to 157)
West Midlands	63	138	(106 to 177)
Mersey	21	102	(63 to 156)
North Western	44	127	(92 to 170)

preventable for the age groups stated. This is typical of variation in clinical practice, resource use, and outcomes seen repeatedly, whether based on routine data, audit, or rigorous research. There may well be valid reasons for some of the values. They need further local investigation and explanation. In some cases they may reflect quality of clinical care.

It is such variation that leads to the kinds of questions raised by the public, policy makers, and managers, illustrated by the newspaper headline above. It is up to the clinical professions to address this issue. There is a belief that clinical care is of the highest quality and offers optimal benefit. The clinical professions must now be able to demonstrate this, not just make claims about it.

Key issues thus are: how can the clinical professions demonstrate the outcome of clinical care? and, how can the clinical professions use information on outcomes to improve care? The ultimate goal is to achieve the greatest potential benefit, in terms of improved health, from available resources. I fully acknowledge the technical difficulties involved but these should be considered challenges, not an excuse for not examining outcomes. I would like to take this forward by going through a series of questions clinicians might ask about outcomes, and issues raised by such questions.

What is the clinical problem?

The first question facing a clinician is to understand the problem presented by the patient. It is becoming increasingly necessary now to extend the scope of this beyond just the clinical features of the problem. For example, for diabetes it is not just blood biochemistry and clinical symptoms and signs that matter. Clinicians are increasingly being required to consider wider aspects such as disability and handicap caused by a clinical disorder; how the patient is able to function; and how patients feel about their situation and its impact on the quality of their life and the lives of their families and carers. Surely it is such broader concerns that should shape the clinical quality agenda. The clinician also needs to consider the severity of the presenting problem and its causes. In many cases, the causes of the presenting problem may be preventable, and the problem may represent a negative outcome of previous care or lack of care.

3

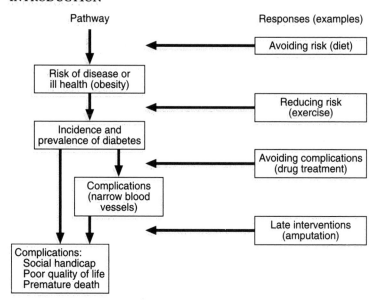

Figure 1.1 Issues in understanding the clinical problem and decision making for non-insulin dependent diabetes

What can the clinician do about the problem?

The decision on what to do should ideally be based on sound research evidence showing that an intervention is likely to lead to a benefit. The scarcity of such research information is well known. An additional concern is that previous research is mostly based on clinical end points and does not show effectiveness in terms of well being or impact on quality of life. In the absence of such research evidence, clinical decision making about intervention tends to be based on judgment and peer opinion. Unfortunately, there isn't always agreement on this, which is a key cause of the observed variation in practice and outcomes. It is now widely acknowledged that individual clinical professionals cannot work in isolation. Most health problems require many professions working together, hence decision making about intervention needs a collaborative approach.

What are the objectives of treatment?

Figure 1.1 presents an overview of the range of issues involved in understanding the clinical problem and making decisions about what to do, for non-insulin dependent diabetes. This figure is in two parts. The left side shows a sequence of events ranging from risk of diabetes, to development of diabetes, its complications, and consequences such as handicap, poor quality of life, and premature death. The right side shows a whole range of clinical actions aimed at influencing different parts of this sequence.

This raises the next clinical question – what are the objectives of treatment? These will obviously vary with the patient's position within this sequence of events. For example, the objective, for someone with a family history of diabetes who is obese, will be the prevention or delay of the onset of diabetes.

Whose perspective?

In arriving at a decision about treatment, clinicians should consider net benefit, given that some treatments have side effects and may even cause harm. In considering such net benefit, clinicians need to take into account a variety of perspectives and concerns of professionals, policy makers, managers, and patients. For example, in the treatment of diabetes with strict diet regimens the clinician may be more concerned about blood sugar levels, the patient more about quality of life. This raises key issues about the extent to which patients are involved in decision making. This aspect will be covered in chapter 4.

What are the services required?

Once the objectives are clear, clinicians may be in a position to specify the interventions, services or treatments. In some cases this may be a single intervention, for example, an operation to amputate a limb – but in many cases a whole range of interventions over time will be required, involving many professionals working in different parts of the NHS and even outside it. The patient may be an active partner in such interventions, particularly so with diabetes.

What are the standards required?

Achievement of the best possible outcomes may depend on delivering services to specified standards. Several initiatives in diabetes care attempt to do this. St Vincent's Joint Task Force is a joint task force between the British Diabetic Association and the Department of Health, to take forward some of the recommendations for improving diabetes services made at a European meeting in St Vincent, Italy, in May 1989.

INTRODUCTION

The Chronic Disease Management Programme is part of the new general practitioner contract and already over 90% of general practitioners have been approved to run chronic disease management programmes. For diabetes, this includes maintaining a register and having clear care and follow up plans and outcome reviews.

A recent report by the Clinical Standards Advisory Group, set up following the NHS reforms, makes several recommendations for standards of diabetes care.

Some of the broader standards that have evolved are a shift of focus from secondary to primary care; that 90% of general practitioners have signed up to quality standards; and recognition of the need to integrate general practitioner and hospital care. The reports also contain some more specific clinical standards.

What are the results?

Once the care is delivered, key questions involve assessing the extent to which the desired results were achieved. The first

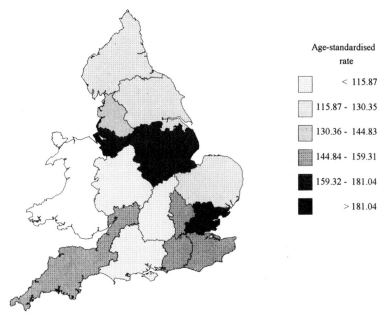

Figure 1.2 Hospital episode rates for ketoacidosis and coma in women, by regional health authority, for year ending 31 March 1990

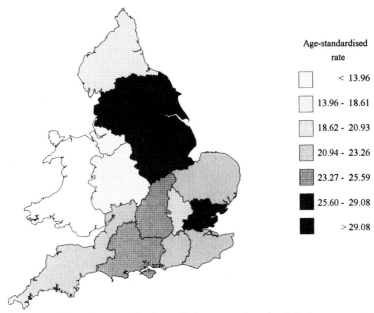

Age-standardised
rate

☐ < 13.96

☐ 13.96 - 18.61

☐ 18.62 - 20.93

☐ 20.94 - 23.26

▨ 23.27 - 25.59

■ 25.60 - 29.08

■ > 29.08

Figure 1.3 Operation rates for lower limb amputations in diabetic women, by regional health authority, for year ending 31 March 1990

question is an audit of the quality of service delivery. Was the service delivered to the standards specified? Such information may suggest that the desired benefit is likely to be achieved, hence it may act as a proxy for future outcome. The second, more important – but more difficult – question is whether the clinical problems changed as expected (for example, control of blood sugar, or weight reduction) and whether this was due to the clinical action. Such attribution is difficult as it needs to take into account other possible influences on health and also allow for the presenting problem and its severity.

This is what we mean by outcome. The Department of Health uses this working definition of health outcome: "attributable effect of intervention or its lack on a previous health state." This is still evolving, and suggestions for improving on it are most welcome.

Figure 1.2 shows regional variation in population rates for hospital admissions due to diabetic ketoacidosis and coma. Figure 1.3 shows similar variation in operation rates for limb amputations associated with diabetes. Once again, there may well be valid reasons for such variation. However, one conclusion is that the NHS is not achieving optimum potential benefit from its diabetes services. The report of the St Vincent's task force recommends improvement in some of these aspects.

How is the Department of Health addressing these issues?

The clinical questions I have just gone through raise a number of important issues that need to be addressed. How are we tackling them?

The Clinical Outcomes Group, which was set up in 1992, chaired jointly by myself and the chief nursing officer, is one national body that has a key role. It was set up to offer advice on the strategic direction of clinical audit and the development of methods to identify and achieve improved outcomes. Its role has evolved and now covers advice on all aspects of quality of clinical care. Its membership embraces a diverse range of disciplines and interests, including the Department of Health, the NHS, health professionals, and patients. There are two lay members representing patients' and the public's perspectives and interests.

The main responsibility for outcomes assessment and its use lies, of course, with the professions. Diabetes care presents a good example of the need to bring a variety of health professionals, different NHS sectors (for example, primary and secondary care), and patients together to tackle the issues. The Department of Health is supporting a range of projects, working closely with the professions, NHS colleagues, and patients to do this. The box lists some of these projects, grouped according to the relevant clinical question. This is just a selection of central initiatives. There are many more. These are described in a leaflet on the work of the department's Central Health Outcomes Unit. These initiatives will not provide all the answers, methods, and systems needed but will gradually take us forward in our thinking and ability to work with outcomes as part of clinical care. A significant result of this enormous set of activities on all fronts is that it has stimulated a more self questioning culture, an important stepping stone for the topic of "outcomes into clinical practice."

Education

There is no point in having all these initiatives if the results do not reach the clinical professions and there is no change in behaviour. The professional education system provides a means of making this happen. This works at several levels: undergraduate education; postgraduate education; continuing education. However, there are some fundamental issues that still need to be addressed. What are the best educational techniques? How do we achieve change in behaviour? Are there any other mechanisms besides education as, for example, financial incentives, status, managerial and contractual requirements? These issues are the subject of ongoing research.

A model for effecting change

I have been through a theoretical framework of issues. However, unless we are able to apply it to the services in practice we are unlikely to achieve the goals I stated earlier. There is a recent initiative that shows that we can actually use outcomes to initiate change in services, leading to better care and, over time, better health. This brings me to the example of cancer. You may recall a report, published recently by the Expert Advisory Group on Cancer, which I chaired. A key premise used by the group to form its recommendation was based on evidence that outcome depends on a critical mass of patients being seen by a clinical team. The information on which this premise was based still needs further development. These are some of the recommendations on appropriate levels of care that were made:

- primary care focus : clarify patterns of referral and follow up;
- designated cancer units in district general hospitals : manage common cancers;
- designated cancer centres : advise on management and treat less common cancers.

Conclusions

In this short space it has been possible to give only an overview of key issues concerning outcomes as part of clinical practice. I wish to highlight the following points:

9

- Information on outcomes, focused around particular clinical questions, is likely to make an important contribution to clinical decision making at the local level;
- Development of such information requires a systematic and structured approach;
- There is a need for such information and intelligence to extend beyond the clinical arena into wider areas such as education and the planning and management of services;
- There is a need for collaboration in the development of methods and systems, in order to avoid duplication of effort;
- There is a substantial collaborative development effort already under way between the Department of Health, the NHS, health professionals, patients, and others.

Summary of Department of Health initiatives likely to contribute to the development of "outcomes" methods and systems

What is the clinical problem?
(Health; severity; determinants)

- Development and review of instruments to measure and value generic and disease specific health states
- Development of National Language of Health
  - Clinical terms projects (coded thesaurus of clinical terms)
  - Health benefit groups
  - Multi-axial classification
- Information management and technology strategy (creation of linked, person based health records)
- Health monitoring
  - Epidemiological overviews
  - Health survey for England and other national surveys
  - Public health common data set
  - Health measurement toolbox
- Central Health Monitoring Unit
- National Health Service Centre for Coding and Classification
- National Casemix Office
- Survey Clearing House (awaiting commission)

What can the clinician do about it? (Information on effectiveness)	• National Health Service Research and Development Strategy • Research into effectiveness/cost-effectiveness of interventions (including Health Technology Assessment) • Health of the Nation Target Effectiveness documents – Coronary heart disease, strokes, etc (forthcoming) • Cost-effectiveness Register (dissemination of pilot version forthcoming) • Effective Health Care Bulletins (7 topics published) • Research Reviews and Dissemination Centre • Cochrane Centre
What are the objectives of treatment?	• Health of the Nation white paper • Local Target Setting – A Discussion Paper • National setting of health objectives and targets • Population health outcomes models • Work on health outcomes indicators
What are the services and standards required?	• Health of the Nation Key Area Handbooks (5 topics) • Health Service Executive letter on clinical effectiveness and guidelines (EL(93)115) • Purchasing for Health (series of speeches) • Epidemiologically Based Needs Assessment Reviews (19 topics) • Development of national guidance on clinical standards • Development of national guidance on service specification

11

What are the results? (Audit of process)	• Development and promotion of medical, nursing, therapy and clinical audit; clinical audit policy • Development of data on interventions: Information Management and Technology Strategy Clinical terms projects (Coded Thesaurus of Clinical Terms) • Development of data on resource use: English health care resource groups • Health service indicators • Audit Information Centre
What are the results? (Audit of outcome)	• Development of health outcome indicators: Population Health Outcome Indicators for the NHS – report of a feasibility study Population Health Outcome Indicators for the NHS – a consultation document • Outcomes audit projects (several) • Confidential Enquiries (maternal deaths, perioperative deaths, stillbirths and deaths in infancy, genetic counselling, suicides and homicides related to mental illness) • Outcomes research projects (several) • Central Health Outcomes Unit • UK Clearing House – Health Outcomes

2 Outcomes research: implications for policy and practice

ALBERT MULLEY

Outcomes research is a relatively new term in the lexicon of clinical and health services research. As such, its meaning is not always clear, particularly when viewed from different vantage points in the health care economy. Doctors, patients, and policy makers have different perceptions and different expectations of outcomes research, and the sum of those expectations constitutes a heavy burden for the fledgling field.[1-5] As we consider how outcomes research can be integrated with clinical practice, and the implications of such an initiative for practice and policy, we should begin with a common understanding of outcomes research and its potential.

Outcomes research can be viewed as the constructive professional response to striking variations in clinical practices including considerable geographic variation in rates of procedures used in seemingly similar populations of patients. Such variations raise disturbing questions about both the cost and the quality of medical care.[6-10] Outcomes research is also a response to equally disturbing variations in clinical outcomes when different providers use the same intervention.[11-13] An important factor in the first issue is accurate information on the relative effectiveness of medical practices. Which treatments work for whom, and when?[14-15] Doctors also need to know more about patients' subjective responses to outcomes of illness and its treatment.

13

Which potentially achievable outcomes are valued by patients, each of whom may bring a unique set of preferences and risk attitudes to a clinical decision?[16–17]

Information about what works and what is valued is essential in determining the right thing to do for a particular patient. The doctor also needs information about how to do it right. This can be derived from an understanding of processes of care, more specifically an understanding of associations between variations in processes and variations in rates of good and bad outcomes. Here, the need for accurate data on processes and outcomes from a range of clinical practices, rather than research settings, is even more compelling. We need to collect and share practice data on what works in medicine and what people value to improve the professional knowledge base; and we need it to provide a scientific basis for "best practice." Outcomes research can provide these data and thereby support professionalism and make quality management tools applicable to clinical care.[9, 18]

What is outcomes research?

Outcomes research refers to the set of activities involved in generating, collecting, analysing, and applying information about the results or outcomes of medical care. At one end of the spectrum is research and development of methods and technologies to measure outcomes of care, including quality of life and functional status among other, more traditional outcomes.

The scientific underpinning of outcomes research derives from empirical studies of the efficacy of medical practices. Examples include prospectively designed studies that vary how care is delivered and document effects on the outcomes of that care (this definition includes clinical trials of alternative treatments or drugs) and studies that observe outcome variations and relate them to differences in the antecedent care (hospital mortality data as a quality of care indicator, for example). Another key and defining data set of outcomes research derives from the study of patient preferences and values concerning the outcomes of care.

Finally, outcomes research uses these data. Indeed, focusing on the outcomes of care to gain insight into the efficacy of medical practice is hardly new. What outcomes research brings to the current health debate is its potential for its integration with clinical practice to improve quality and efficiency throughout a health care system.

Uses of outcomes research

- For the individual physician and patient making a clinical decision, outcomes research can accurately predict patient specific outcomes based on the collective experience of the medical profession with other patients.
- Outcomes research provides objective information on patients' preferences, enhancing their potential role in clinical decision making.
- Data revealing how people value alternative outcomes can inform resource allocation and other policy decisions – for example, using aggregate measures of benefits to make purchasing decisions which improve allocation efficiencies.
- Comparative outcomes data generated by providers can be used to identify best practice and develop practice guidelines and to distinguish between practice variation which is appropriate and desirable, and practice variation which is not.
- Perhaps most significant for improving quality of care, rigorous comparison of outcomes across providers and processes of care supports the profession, updating continuously its knowledge base to provide a scientific basis for professional self assessment and improvement.

Outcomes research and clinical decisions: the case of benign prostatic hyperplasia

The potential of outcomes research in clinical practice can best be understood by considering a particular clinical decision: in this case, what to do for patients with benign prostatic hyperplasia.[16,17,19] This condition afflicts most older men. Like many other conditions, it compromises the quality of life, which may be made better by one or more therapeutic interventions. Transurethral prostatectomy is performed at highly variable rates in the United States and the United Kingdom, often with highly variable outcomes.[19,20] Consider the case of a married, sexually active 72 year old man with increasing symptoms of bladder irritation and bladder outlet obstruction due to benign prostatic hyperplasia. His primary care physician refers him to a urologist, who recommends surgery – a transurethral prostatectomy

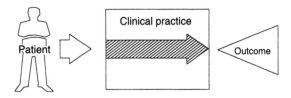

Figure 2.1 A patient with a certain health state – symptoms of benign prostatic hyperplasia – has a clinical encounter. The square represents the structural elements of practice; the embedded arrow represents the process of care. The three sides of the triangle represent the physical, psychological, and social dimensions of the outcome. For the purposes of outcomes research, the health outcome is that change in health status or patient wellbeing that can be attributed to the antecedent care

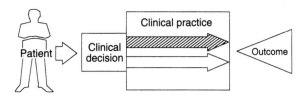

Figure 2.2 The parallel arrows indicate alternative processes of care, either of which produce an outcome. The choice among alternatives requires a clinical decision

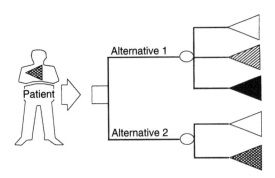

Figure 2.3 A simple decision model. The decision, a choice between alternative 1 (TURP) and alternative 2 (watchful waiting) is represented by the square nodes. Uncertain outcomes contingent on each treatment are represented by the triangles; for the patient with benign prostatic hyperplasia the white triangle represents symptom relief, the light triangle represents loss of sexual function, the black triangle represents operative mortality. With alternative 2, the patient may experience symptom relief, but, more likely, his symptoms, represented by the dark triangle, will persist

(TURP) – to remove some prostate tissue around the urethra, thereby alleviating the obstruction. However, there are alternatives. The patient could take one of several new medical treatments in an effort to relieve symptoms, or he could do nothing but monitor the situation with the help of his doctor, a strategy we might call "watchful waiting." Clinical practice inevitably involves choosing among such alternative processes of care, for which the results are uncertain, and for each alternative there are multiple possible outcomes. Consider the patient's choice between surgery and "watchful waiting." If he chooses surgery there is some probability of relief of symptoms; there is also some probability of surgical complications (permanent urinary or sexual dysfunction, or death). The outcome of "watchful waiting" is also uncertain: his symptoms may improve spontaneously or may persist, or complications such as acute urinary retention may occur. To make an informed decision, our patient and his doctor need to know the estimated probabilities of these different outcomes for alternative treatments.

The determinants of these probabilities are several. Firstly, different patients face different outcome probabilities – a function of their disease severity, comorbidity, and other variables that affect prognosis. Secondly, differences in how alternative therapies are applied and how their outcomes are measured are equally significant. Therefore, to estimate outcome probabilities accurately requires the characterisation of patients (including demographic variables, disease severity, and comorbidity conditions) and systematic application of alternative treatments and outcome measurement.

The most accurate outcome probability estimates for our patient derive from the collective outcomes experience of similar men who under similar conditions chose either transurethral prostatectomy or "watchful waiting."[20] Ideally, a randomised trial would have been conducted among patients just like the patient at hand. But many clinical problems have not been evaluated by trials. Even when trial results are available they often apply to a narrow range of patients seen in clinical practice. Outcomes measured in trials may not be those that are of most concern to patients. Furthermore, trial results may be less than robust, as therapeutic interventions evolve as a result of continuous refinement in both medical and surgical interventions. Outcomes research includes prospective observational trials that aggregate, define, and organise outcomes data, and

17

in so doing outcomes research provides individual doctors with outcomes data derived from the ongoing collective clinical experience of the profession.

Yet even the most accurate outcome probabilities are not sufficient for informed clinical decision making. Patients' preferences also play a role in determining the right thing to do. Consider, for example, how patients with benign prostatic hyperplasia who face the same outcome probabilities might value them differently. For example, we can assume that virtually all patients would feel best about symptom improvement and worst about death. However, they might assign very different relative values to other possible outcomes, including urinary dysfunction (or its relief) and sexual function (or its compromise). Well informed clinical decisions must consider these preferences. If they do not, we run the risk of providing treatment to patients who do not value the expected outcome while withholding it from those who do. In other words, if individual clinical decisions rely on the preferences of a hypothetical "average" patient, then efficient allocation of resources is at risk. In a prospective study of men well informed about treatment options for benign prostatic hyperplasia, the relative values regarding symptoms and sexual function were the most important determinants of choice.[20, 21]

Aggregate data on preference also provide valuable information. On the one hand, these data help inform patients' value judgments; on the other, they help doctors recognise and accommodate those preferences and their variability. The sequences of figures 2.4–2.10 illustrate this two way feedback

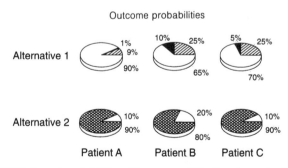

Figure 2.4 Estimated probabilities of outcomes following alternative 1 (TURP) and alternative 2 (watchful waiting) for three different patients (see figure 2.3 for key)

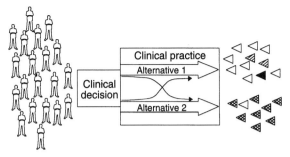

Figure 2.5 Individual decisions are made for multiple patients with similar conditions. Their outcomes can serve as a source of information for estimating outcome probabilities

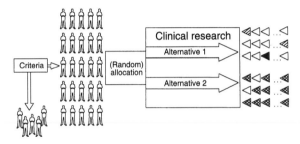

Figure 2.6 Clinical research as a source of outcome probability estimates. Inclusion and exclusion criteria are used to make the patient group homogeneous

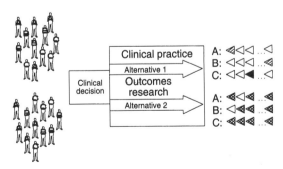

Figure 2.7 Outcomes research requires careful characterisation of patients with demographic variables and measures of disease severity and comorbid conditions. It also requires systematic measurement of outcomes

19

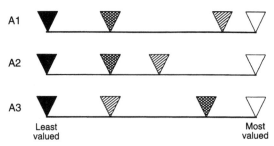

Value judgments for 3 patients

A1

A2

A3

Least valued — Most valued

Figure 2.8 Three patients who face the same probabilities of outcomes have different relative preferences. The black triangle represents death, the light shading represents sexual dysfunction, the dark shading represents persistent urinary symptoms, and the white represents relief of symptoms

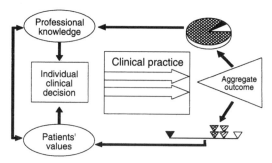

Figure 2.9 A dual feedback loop with aggregate outcomes informing both professional estimates of outcome probabilities and patients' value judgments

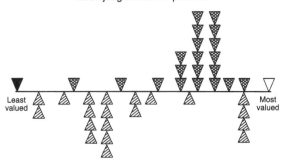

Value judgments in n patients

Least valued — Most valued

Figure 2.10 A hypothetical distribution of responses to questions about the relative value of urinary symptoms (above the line) and sexual dysfunction (below the line)

loop. The pie diagram (see figure 2.4) represents the outcome probability estimates that can be continuously improved by the ongoing aggregation of collective clinical experience. The triangles on the linear scales reflect patients' subjective responses to outcomes. Feedback of this information can provide a basis for current patients to better anticipate what life will be like when transformed by illness or alternative treatments, thereby helping them make more informed choices.

Outcomes research also yields comparative outcomes data on different providers, different applications of the "same" processes of care, and different resource inputs. Indeed, just as patients differ greatly, providers differ greatly in how they assemble and apply processes of care, and these differences may affect clinical outcomes.

Systematically collected comparative data on outcomes and processes would have a profound impact on decision making throughout the health care system. Identifying what is most effective in diagnosing and treating illnesses would enable the medical profession continuously to improve its knowledge base and the quality of its care. It would enable patients to assume a more informed role in health care decisions and would provide purchasers with a scientific basis for selecting among providers and evaluating medical claims. Comparative data linking resource inputs to outcomes would identify opportunities to achieve greater efficiencies in delivery of care. These elements of an outcomes research system are illustrated in figures 2.11–2.14.

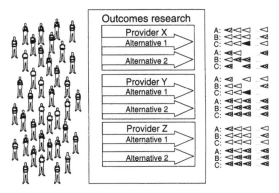

Figure 2.11 To meet its potential in making collective clinical experience a source of probability estimates, outcomes research requires standardised baseline and outcome measures, by multiple providers

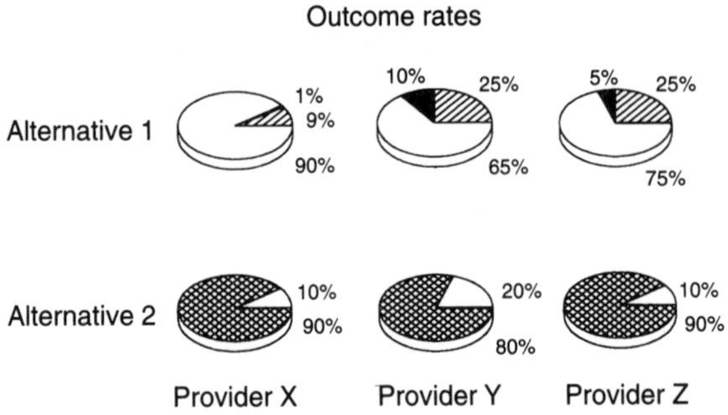

Outcome rates

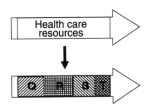

Alternative 1

1%
9%
90%

10% 25%
65%

5% 25%
75%

Alternative 2

10%
90%

20%
80%

10%
90%

Provider X   Provider Y   Provider Z

Figure 2.12 Comparative outcome rates for the same interventions used by different providers

Health care
resources

Figure 2.13 Different inputs (hospital, day nursing time, laboratory services, etc) are combined to comprise a therapeutic intervention

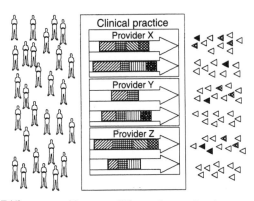

Clinical practice
Provider X

Provider Y

Provider Z

Figure 2.14 Different providers use different inputs for the same therapeutic interventions

Note that one therapeutic alternative may be participation in a randomised trial. Patients who opt for randomisation could be followed along with those who do not.

Outcomes research can also inform policy decisions. In brief, by providing information about the choices patients make when knowledgeable about outcome probabilities, outcomes research can inform investment decisions and improve the efficiency of resource allocation in terms of treatment alternatives, treatment rates, and the value obtained by patients.

Outcomes research and clinical decisions: the dimensions of the problem and opportunity

Benign prostatic hyperplasia is a striking example of the potential value of outcomes research for several reasons. Relatively little clinical research had been done in the area before it became the target of those concerned about practice variation and the underlying professional uncertainty. Treatment decisions about other high variation conditions, such as low back pain and benign conditions of the uterus, are made in the face of similar collective professional uncertainty. There is great potential for outcomes research here too.

However, the potential of outcomes research, as described above, is not limited to these relatively unstudied conditions. Coronary artery bypass graft surgery may be one of the most studied surgical procedures. Three major randomised trials and several smaller trials were conducted during the 1970s.[22–24] But no trial or series of trials is applicable to all patients for whom this treatment may be used, nor can they provide lasting answers to relevant clinical questions as technology advances. When eligibility criteria from the three major trials were applied to the population of patients in the Duke database for whom bypass surgery was a consideration, approximately 90% of the patients on the database would have been ineligible for the trials.[25] Since the trials were completed, there have been dramatic advances in surgical technique (for example, cold cardioplegia, which allows more extensive revascularisation, and internal mammary artery implants, which extend the duration of effective revascularisation). There have also been dramatic advances in alternative treatments as medical treatment has progressed and angioplasty has been introduced and refined. Wide disagreement between those developing guidelines for coronary artery bypass grafting in the United States and Britain underscores the continuing uncertainty as well as the influence of implicit value judgments in such processes.[26] Though we need randomised trials, we cannot afford to squander the new knowledge that can be gleaned from disciplined, systematic aggregation of ongoing collective clinical experience.

Another example of a clinical condition that could benefit from this approach is breast cancer. Like coronary disease and its treatment, it has been extensively studied.[27–29] Primary treatment of the disease is not subject to demand induced by suppliers, yet there is a great deal of variation in treatment approaches, reflecting differences in professional opinion.[30–33] The strength with which these opinions are held, in favour of either mastectomy or lumpectomy followed by irradiation, often precludes truly informed choice by the women who live with the consequences. There is evidence that women can make these choices, and that whether or not they have the opportunity to do so is a determinant of important outcomes, including their psychological response to the illness and its treatment.[34–35]

Our need for better information about what works and what is valued, and about how to do it right, is a general one. Few conditions would not be better treated if we developed a system of outcomes research that could be brought into clinical practice. Systematic examination of those outcomes that are most important to patients would improve the quality of medical decisionmaking. Associations between variable rates of achieving those outcomes with variable processes would improve the quality of care.

Moving outcomes into clinical practice: implementation challenges

Technological limitations remain a challenge, particularly our ability to assess patients' preferences and to control for disease severity. Other issues relate to the resources required for outcomes research: who will do the work; who will pay for it; and who will audit the data and assure its integrity. There is, however, progress. Systems have been developed that help clinicians manage the professional knowledge base and make it understandable for patients. Shared decisionmaking programmes provide patient specific outcome probability estimates while capturing patients' defining characteristics for enrollment in

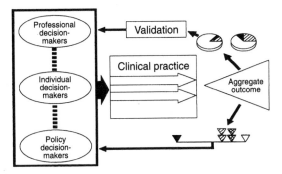

Figure 2.15 A conceptual model of outcomes research with information about outcome probabilities and comparable outcome rates, as well as patients' values and informed choices among alternative interventions made available to providers, patients, and policy makers

either randomised trials or prospective cohort studies. The same programmes provide patients with vicarious experience in the form of video testimonials from previous patients who have made treatment choices and experienced good and bad outcomes. Already, a shared decisionmaking programme for men with benign prostate hyperplasia has been shown to have a significant effect on treatment choice. Equally important, it has served to assemble the largest available cohort of men with the condition, thereby refining our understanding of the clinical course of benign prostatic hyperplasia, as well as response to treatment.[36, 37, 38]

Doctors, at least initially, respond ambivalently to the collection and sharing of outcomes information. On the one hand, it offers a constructive response to evident problems of professional knowledge – an opportunity to develop a system that will support the profession by continuously updating its information base and providing comparative rates for benchmarking and continuous improvement of care. On the other hand, there is a perception among some doctors that outcomes data will lead to practice guidelines which will require them to surrender their judgments to "cookbook medicine."   .

Perhaps more troublesome are the issues relating to the data themselves: who "owns" them, who validates them, and who controls their interpretation. Identifying mechanisms to validate outcomes data and protect practitioners and other providers against its misuse must be a priority for all involved.

IMPLICATIONS FOR POLICY AND PRACTICE

A new vehicle for constructive change in health care is long overdue, and the potential of outcomes research to set the direction for this change is clear. It shifts the focus away from external regulation and inspection in favour of professionalism and internal improvement. It adopts an aggressive regard for patients' preferences and for their role in clinical decisionmaking. It seeks to generate new knowledge from clinical practice and make that information available to providers in a timely fashion to improve care. Finally, it is grounded in an explicit commitment to improving quality and value in health care.

This work was supported by the Pew Charitable Trusts and the Agency for Health Care Policy and Research. I thank David Blumenthal for his contribution to an earlier draft of this manuscript.

1 Wennberg J, Gittelsohn A. Small area variations in health care delivery. *Science* 1973; **182**: 1102–8.
2 Wennberg JE, Gittelsohn A. Variations in medical care among small areas. *Sci Am* 1982; **246**: 120–34.
3 Chassin MR, Brook RH, Park RE, Keesey J, Fink A, Kosecoff J, *et al*. Variations in the use of medical and surgical services by the Medicare population. *N Engl J Med* 1986; 314: 285–90.
4 Chassin MR, Kosecoff J, Park RE, Winslow CM, Kahn KL, Merrick NJ, *et al*. Does inappropriate use explain geographic variations in the use of health care services? *JAMA* 1987; **258**: 2533–7.
5 Bunker JP. Variations in hospital admissions and the appropriateness of care: American preoccupations? *BMJ* 1990; **301**: 531–2.
6 Wenneker MB, Epstein AM. Racial inequalities in the use of procedures for patients with ischemic heart disease in Massachusetts. *N Engl J Med* 1989; : 253–7.
7 Greenfield S, Blanco DM, Elashoff RM, Ganz PA. Patterns of care related to age of breast cancer patients. *JAMA* 1987; **257**: 2766–70.
8 Held PJ, Pauly MV, Boubjerg JD, Newmann J, Salvateira. Access to transplantation: has the United States eliminated income and racial differences? *Arch Intern Med* 1988; **748**: 2594–600.
9 Institute of Medicine. *Medicare: a strategy for quality assurance*. Vol 1. Washington DC: National Academy Press, 1990.
10 Wennberg JE, Barnes BA, Zubkoff M. Professional uncertainty and the problem of supplier-induced demand. *Soc Sci Med* 1982; **16**: 811–42.
11 Showstack JA, Rosenfeld KE, Garnick DW, Luft HS, Schaffarzick RW, Fowles J. Association of volume with outcome of coronary artery bypass graft surgery. *JAMA* 1987; **257**: 785–9.
12 Wennberg JE, Roos N, Sola L, Schori A, Jaffe R. Use of claims data systems to evaluate health care outcomes: mortality and reoperation following prostatectomy. *JAMA* 1987; **257**: 933–6.
13 Hannan EL, O'Donnell JF, Kilburn H, Bernard HR, Yazici A. Investigation of the relationship between volume and mortality for surgical procedures performed in New York state hospitals. *JAMA* 1989; **262**: 503–10.
14 Roper WL, Winkenwerder W, Hackbarth GM, Krakauer H. Effectiveness in health care. An initiative to evaluate and improve medical practice. *N Engl J Med* 1988; **319**: 1197–202.
15 Wennberg JE. Dealing with medical practice variations: a proposal for action. *Health Affairs* 1984; **3**: 6-32.
16 Mulley AG. Medical decision making and practice variation. In: Anderson and Mooney eds. *The challenges of medical practice variations*. London: MacMillan, 1990.

17 Mulley AG. Assessing patients' utilities: can the ends justify the means? *Med Care* 1989; 27: S269–81.
18 Berwick DM. Continuous improvement as an ideal in health care. *N Engl J Med* 1989; 320: 53–6.
19 Wennberg JE, Mulley AG Jr, Hanley D, Timothy RP, Fowler FJ Jr, Roos NP, *et al.* An assessment of prostatectomy for benign urinary tract obstruction. Geographic variations and the evaluation of medical care outcomes. *JAMA* 1988; 259: 3027–30.
20 Barry MJ. Medical outcomes research and benign prostatic hyperplasia. *The Prostate* 1990; 3: S61–74.
21 Fowler FJ, Wennberg JE, Timothy RP, Barry MJ, Mulley AG, Hanley D. Symptom status and quality of life following prostatectomy. *JAMA* 1988; 259: 3018–22.
22 Veterans Administration Coronary Artery Bypass Surgery Cooperative Study Group. Eleven-year survival in the veterans administration randomized trial of coronary bypass surgery for stable angina. *N Engl J Med* 1984; 311: 1333–9.
23 European Coronary Surgery Study Group. Long-term results of prospective randomized study of coronary bypass surgery for stable angina pectoris. *Lancet* 1982; ii: 1173–80.
24 CASS Principal Investigators. Myocardial infarction and survival in the CASS randomized trial. *N Engl J Med* 1984; 310: 750–8.
25 Hlatky MA, Califf RM, Harrell FE, Lee KL, Mark DB, Pryor DB. Comparison of predictions based on observational data with the results of randomized controlled clinical trials of coronary bypass surgery. *JACC* 1988; 11: 237–45.
26 Mulley AG, Eagle KA. What is inappropriate care? *JAMA* 1988; 260: 540–1.
27 Veronesi U, Saccozzi R, Del Vecchio M, Banfi A, Clemente C, De Lena M, *et al.* Comparing radical mastectomy with quadrantectomy, axillary dissection and radiotherapy in patients with small cancers of the breast. *N Engl J Med* 1981; 305: 6–11.
28 Fisher B, Redmond C, Poisson R, Margolese R, Wolmark N, Wickerham L, *et al.* Eight-year results of a randomized clinical trial comparing total mastectomy and lumpectomy with or without irradiation in the treatment of breast cancer. *N Engl J Med* 1989; 320: 822–8.
29 Early Breast Cancer Trialists' Collaborative Group. Systemic treatment of early breast cancer by hormonal, cytotoxic, or immune therapy. *Lancet* 1992; 339: 1–15, 71–85.
30 Farrow DC, Hunt WC, Samet JM. Geographic variation in the treatment of localized breast cancer. *N Engl J Med* 1992; 326: 1097–101.
31 Nattinger AB, Gottlieb MS, Veum J, Yahnke D, Goodwin JS. Geographic variation in the use of breast-conserving treatment for breast cancer. *N Engl J Med* 1992; 326: 1102–7.
32 Tarbox B, Rockwood J, Abernathy C. Are modified radical mastectomies done for T1 breast cancer because of surgeon's advice or patient's choice? *Am J Surg* 1992; 164: 417–22.
33 GIVIO (Interdisciplinary Group for Cancer Care Evaluation). Survey of treatment of primary breast cancer in Italy. *Br J Cancer* 1988; 57: 630–4.
34 Wilson RG, Hart A, Dawes PJDK. Mastectomy or conservation: the patient's choice. *BMJ* 1988; 297: 1167–9.
35 Morris T, Ingham R. Choice of surgery for early breast cancer: psychosocial considerations. *Soc Sci Med* 1988; 27: 1257–62.
36 Mulley AG. Applying effectiveness and outcomes research to clinical practice. In: Heithoff KA, Lohr KN, eds. *Effectiveness and outcomes in health care.* Washington, DC: National Academy Press, 1990.
37 Kasper JF, Mulley AG Jr, Wennberg JE. Developing shared decision-making programs to improve the quality of health care. *Quality Rev Bull* 1992; : 183–90.
38 Barry MJ, Fowler FJ, Mulley AG Jr, Henderson JV Jr, Wennberg JE. Patient reactions to a program designed to facilitate patient participation in treatment decisions for benign prostatic hyperplasia. *Med Care* (in press)

3 Clinical teams, general practice, audit, and outcomes

IRENE HIGGINSON

Although outcome measurement of hospital based and acute inpatient and outpatient services is fairly well developed,[1,2] outcome measurement in community teams and general practice is often still in its early stages. There are four main reasons for this. Firstly, measures already developed for hospital based services may not be directly applicable for general practice. The development of new measures or the adaptation of existing measures in general practice or community settings requires fairly extensive preliminary testing, which can be lengthy.

Secondly, there is no single common intervention of community teams or of general practice. Instead their work tends to involve many different interventions, which have quite different goals – for example, treating a leg ulcer, managing a patient with diabetes, assessing and referring a patient with a cataract. Health outcome is defined as "any end result which is attributable to a health service intervention."[3] Thus, the outcomes need to be sensitive to the specific health service intervention, and when there are multiple interventions it is important to have outcomes that will reflect each different intervention.

Thirdly, community teams and general practice tend to involve a multidisciplinary input, which has often not been reflected in hospital based measurements. Finally, some of the areas of care

---

Box 1 – Potential uses for outcome measures in community teams and general practice

- Clinical audit
- Evaluation
- Maintaining quality
- Purchasing
- Targeting service better
- Improving clinical assessment and monitoring

---

may include the assessment of patients who are extremely frail or confused and who may not be able to complete self assessment forms.[4] In some instances, the views of the carer have been used, but this is appropriate only when a carer exists, and for an increasing proportion of elderly people this is no longer the case. Also, the views of a carer may conflict with those of the patient.[5]

Despite these constraints, it is possible to develop outcome measures for community teams and in general practice, and these measures have a number of uses. The potential uses for outcome measurement in this setting are shown in box 1. This paper provides examples of outcome measurement in palliative care and in dementia care, illustrating their use in these areas and highlighting some of the difficulties in developing measures.

Approach to outcome development in palliative care

Our study, carried out in five units in the South East of England, aimed to develop outcome measures for community teams which cared for patients with advanced cancer. The teams were multidisciplinary and consisted of nurses (Macmillan nurses), usually one or two doctors, a social worker, occasionally a chaplain, an occupational therapist, and a physiotherapist or dietician. These teams work within defined catchment areas and assist and advise on the care of patients with advanced cancer who may need extra support because of troublesome symptoms, emotional or family concerns, or practical needs or during the final stage of life. The teams work alongside existing professionals such as the general practitioner or district nurse, offering shared

29

Box 2 – Criteria for measures of outcome

Validity – does the instrument measure what it intends to measure? This can include content, face, criterion and construct validity.

Reliability – does the instrument produce consistent results when used on the same population?

Responsiveness to change – can the instrument detect clinically meaningful changes?

Appropriateness of format – is the instrument suitable for its intended use?

---

care to assist, advise, and support the existing professionals. The staff of the teams are normally highly trained in managing symptoms and alleviating emotional problems. They also often have a role in coordinating services and in providing skilled communication with the patient and family.[6, 7]

Review of the literature indicated that there were few measures for palliative care.[8] Measures that had been used, adapted from cancer treatment trials, had been heavily criticised and were not found to be responsive to changes in clinical practice.[9] Our criteria for any measure are shown in box 2 – these are adapted from those used in standard texts.[1, 10] We found that most measures had been shown to have some degree of validity and reliability. However, responsiveness to clinical change was rarely tested. Furthermore, most measures were developed for use in research studies, had not been tested in community settings, were lengthy, and required extra trained staff to administer them.

To develop outcomes for palliative care we worked initially with one community team and expanded this to five teams to develop the Support Team Assessment Schedule to reflect more closely the outcomes of palliative care.[11] This schedule consists of 17 items, 10 concerned with the patient and family and seven with service provision, as shown in box 3. The items cover physical, psychosocial, communication, spiritual, and health service domains, as well as family concerns (because the patient and family are the unit of care) and the need for future planning (making a will, for example) as desired by the patient.[11]

Definitions for each item were agreed and followed a 0 (best) to 4 (worst) rating scale. To enhance reliability the individual ratings

---

Box 3 – The Support Team Assessment Schedule (STAS)

Patient and family* items:
Pain control
Symptom control
Patient anxiety
Family anxiety
Patient insight
Family insight
Planning
Predictability
Spiritual
Communication between patient and family

Service items:
Practical aid
Financial
Wasted time
Communication between professionals[†]
Communication of professionals to patient and family
Advising professionals
Professional anxiety

* Family = nearest carer or significant other.
† Professionals = other than the teams involved in the care.

---

were made as specific and clear as possible. An example is shown in box 4. Full details of all definitions have been published.[11]

Analysis of the content, face, criterion, and construct validity of the schedule showed that the areas covered were acceptable to teams and patients, that professional ratings were reasonably well correlated and showed reasonable agreement with patient and family ratings, and that contemporary ratings according to the

---

Box 4 – Definition of one item in Support Team Assessment Schedule: Pain Control

Effect of the pain on the patient:

0 = None
1 = Occasional or grumbling single pain; patient is not bothered to be rid of symptom
2 = Moderate distress, occasional bad days; pain limits some activity possible within extent of disease
3 = Severe pain present often; activities and concentration markedly affected by pain
4 = Severe and continuous overwhelming pain; unable to think of other matters

---

schedule were correlated with those of a quality of life measure for patients who were early in care.[11-13] Reliability testing using simulated patients with paired and multiple grouped scorings, including the range of professionals (doctors, nurses, and social workers), showed good reliability for 16 out of 17 items.[11] One item, predictability (indicating the need to provide prognostic information), was not found to be reliable and has been removed from the schedule. Given that professionals are usually inaccurate in providing prognostic estimates,[14] it was not surprising that this item was unreliable.

Teams agree methods of recording, depending on their circumstances. Most often, a team will record assessments weekly; their clinical records are adapted to include this information.[11, 15] The schedule was found to be responsive to clinical change and increases or reductions in score could be mapped back prior to events. An example of one woman's score is shown in box 5 and figure 3.1.

The Support Team Assessment Schedule was also found to be an appropriate format. On average, assessments could be completed in two minutes per patient. Therefore, although workload was increased, many teams felt that the benefits outweighed the extra time involved. The schedule was found to be clinically useful as a tool for improving communication about a patient's condition between team members and in monitoring the

---

Box 5 – Scores on Support Team Assessment Schedule for one patient

This represents the scores of a 67 year old woman with a squamous cell carcinoma of the lung who was receiving ifosfamide chemotherapy. On referral to the support teams she had moderate problems of symptom control, especially pain and anxiety, and vomiting. Her pain and vomiting were controlled by using a subcutaneous infusion of medication and she was discharged home. She was subsequently readmitted for chemotherapy, and the rise in score was related to her extreme fear and anxiety before each course of treatment. Following discharge and through the support team's care, her symptoms and anxiety again improved and her problems remained low throughout the few weeks until her death at home.

Reproduced by kind permission of the editors of *Palliative Medicine*.[16]

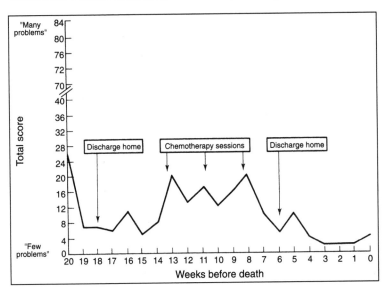

Figure 3.1   Total score on Support Team Assessment Schedule for one patient. (Reproduced by kind permission of the editors of *Palliative Medicine*,[16] published by Edward Arnold.)

change of individual patients during care. It also helped new team members learn more about the aspects that should be included within a palliative care assessment, and help team members to review patient care.[11]

Results of using the outcomes measure

Results from using this outcome measure to audit the work of palliative care teams have shown improvements for many patients in most of the aspects of care but also some failings which required attention.[11, 15] Examples of the results are shown in box 6.

In addition to showing which aspects were or were not improved, use of the schedule was also able to detect where assessments were missed. For example, hospital based teams less frequently recorded assessments related to the family's needs. This included the items "family anxiety" and "family insight."[11] Spiritual assessments were assessed late in 29% of patients and never assessed in a further 48%.[15] As a result of some of these

33

Box 6 – Main findings from palliative care audit

- Teams were able to show effectiveness in many areas
- Family needs were not being assessed by some hospital based teams
- Family anxiety was difficult to alleviate, but family members most at risk of high anxiety could be identified
- Although pain was well controlled, shortness of breath was often not controlled
- Late referrals had more problems and needed much work in a short time
- Spiritual assessments were often missed by some teams

---

findings, teams attempted to develop clinical algorithms to predict those patients who would have the most severe problems or symptoms – for example, uncontrolled breathlessness or severe anxiety in the family.

Future developments

Although the Support Team Assessment Schedule was initially developed for use in clinical audit, it has been used in effectiveness studies.[15] It is currently being tested and adapted for use with patients with HIV/AIDS who have advanced disease,[11] in general community nursing settings, in inpatient hospices and day care,[17] and in general practice. The project in general practice (box 7) is in the early stages of planning; pilot funding has been identified from the Cancer Relief Macmillan Fund.

The schedule is also being adapted and used in other countries and has been translated into Italian, Spanish, Catalan, Dutch, Flemish, and Canadian-English.

Approach to outcomes development for dementia care

A study in inner London aimed to identify and evaluate potential outcome measures for use with specialist community services for people with dementia. The project was based in

---

Box 7 – Adaptation of STAS for use in general practice

Setting:
- Rural practice – 3.5 general practitioners
- 35% of patients over 65 years of age
- 17 bed community hospital

Objectives:
- To agree aspects of primary care work to be included and identify which items of the schedule can be used and where new items are needed
- To develop and pilot the adapted measure for its appropriateness, utility, and speed of completion
- To record data on patients who need palliative care; analyse results; test responsiveness, reliability, face validity

Output from project:
- Potential measure, ready for more detailed testing

Kensington and Chelsea, and Westminster Health Authority, in which three different services, operating within defined catchment areas, offer extra support for people with dementia and for their families. Two of these are community teams and include doctors, community psychiatric nurses, a psychologist, occupational therapists, and social workers. They accept referrals from general practitioners, hospital staff, social workers, and a variety of other professionals. The third service – the Admiral Nursing service – provides support for the carers of elderly people with dementia and consists of two full time clinical nurse specialists.[18]

The project had two phases. A systematic review of the literature identified potential outcome measures, which were evaluated according to predetermined criteria of validity, reliability, responsiveness to change, and appropriateness of format (see box 2). Then, to prioritise the objectives of specialist community services for people with dementia, a questionnaire was sent to specialist teams, general practitioners, district nurses, and carers. All stages of the project were presented to a project advisory committee, which consisted of a psychiatrist of old age, a nurse caring for elderly people with dementia, a purchaser, a carer, a relevant scientist, and the study team. The shortlisted measures were also discussed with three local services.

Results of the literature review and questionnaire survey of dementia care

The literature review identified 81 scales, which were assessed according to the standard criteria. In three studies patient assessment scales had been used to determine the outcome of community services; two had been unable to detect differences between groups receiving different services, and the remaining study was uncontrolled. More studies had used carer based measures to evaluate the provision of health services, but only four measures had been able to show changes in the carers of people with dementia. Therefore, although no patient based measures and only four of the carer based measures had previously been successfully used to measure the outcome of community services, we were able to draw up a shortlist of measures with potential for further testing. Within the shortlist were nine out of 58 (15%) measures relevant to the dementia sufferer, and nine out of 23 (39%) relevant to the informal carer.[19]

The questionnaire was sent to 33 members of specialist community teams caring for people with dementia, 18 primary care staff, and seven carers or ex-carers of dementia sufferers (the same questionnaire was used by an interviewer with the carers). In all, 44/51 (86%) of professionals and all seven (100%) carers responded. The priority objectives are shown in box 8.

The three groups of respondents differed slightly in their priorities for specialist services. Primary care workers were more likely than specialist team members to prioritise the needs of other non-specialist staff and the physical health of the sufferer and the carer. The only major difference between carers and specialist providers was in carers' low ranking of aims to reduce the

---

Box 8 – Priority objectives for specialist community services for people with dementia

- To improve psychological wellbeing, maintain social functioning, and ensure safety of the sufferer
- To improve psychological wellbeing, improve knowledge and skill, maximise satisfaction, and improve social functioning of the carer
- To improve coordination between services

Box 9 – Possible outcome measures for community services for dementia

Brief Assessment Schedule
Rapid Disability Rating Scale-2
Cornell Scale
Behaviour and Mood Disturbance Scale
Alzheimer's Deficit Scale
Perceived Stress Scale
Caregiver Appraisal
Support Team Assessment Schedule
Gilleard's Problem Checklist

Ramsay M, Winget C, Higginson I. *Personal communication*

---

sufferer's inappropriate behaviour. This last finding surprised us, because inappropriate behaviour is cited as the major source of distress to carers. After comparison of the shortlist of measures from the literature review with the important objectives, the scales shown in box 9 were recommended for further testing and possible use of outcome measures for specialist community services for people with dementia.

Discussion

Both of these studies have limitations, which are described in more detail elsewhere.[11-13, 18, 19] Firstly, attempting to define the objectives of the services was often difficult. Many health professionals continue to regard their work more in terms of process (making an assessment, offering treatment) rather than outcome (improving the mental health of the patient or carer). Secondly, none of the samples of professionals or patients or carers included in the studies were randomly selected. When considering the services, we concentrated on all the staff in a few services, and we cannot be certain that their views can be extrapolated to other areas of the country, where conditions may be different. Information from carers and patients was subject to similar bias and limited to those patients and carers whom we could interview. However, review of the literature does not indicate that there are substantial differences between our findings and those in other areas of the country or among other groups of patients and carers. Finally, we do not believe that any of the measures described would reflect the entire work of the community teams. For example, the Support Team Assessment Schedule does not include the educational work of palliative teams or their follow up during bereavement. The development of these measures represents the first, quite large, step in developing measures for community services, which hitherto had been largely unavailable.

Such development needs collaboration between those providing the services and the purchasers of health care. To facilitate this process we have begun to introduce a requirement to include outcomes assessment as part of their work in the contract between Kensington and Chelsea and Westminster Health Authority and our local providers. We have developed a separate section of the contract to deal with the provider's work towards Health of the Nation targets, audit, and health outcomes. The task is not intended to be onerous. In the area of health outcomes, providers are only required to show they are developing the measurement of outcomes in one or two areas through joint agreement with ourselves. Progress is monitored in separate meetings between the relevant providers and representatives from the public health and purchasing departments; so far they have included the use of a standardised depression scale for health visitors to monitor post natal depression, the use of the Support Team Assessment Schedule in the hospital setting, the audit of a new mental health assessment service, and continence outcomes.

1 Wilkin D, Hallm L, Doggett MA. *Measures of need and outcome for primary health care.* Oxford: Oxford University Press, 1992.
2 Hopkins A. *Measuring the outcomes of medical care.* London: Royal College of Physicians, 1990.
3 Department of Health. *On the state of the public health: the annual report of the chief medical officer for the year 1991.* London: HMSO, 1992.
4 Cartwright A, Seal C. *The natural history of a survey: an account of the methodological issues encountered in a study of life before death.* London: King Edward's Hospital Fund, 1990.
5 Higginson I, Priest P, McCarthy M. Are bereaved families a valid proxy for a patient's assessment of dying? *Soc Sci Med* 1994; 38: 553–7.
6 Evans C, McCarthy M. Referral and survival of patients accepted by a terminal care support team. *J Epidemiol Community Health* 1984; 38: 310–4.
7 Hockley JM, Dunlop R, Davies RJ. Survey of distressing symptoms in dying patients and their families in hospital and the response to a symptom control team. *BMJ* 1988; 296: 1715–7.
8 Higginson I, McCarthy M. Evaluation of palliative care: steps to quality assurance? *Palliative Medicine* 1989; 3: 267–74.
9 Mount BM, Scott JF. Whither hospice evaluation? *J Chron Disease* 1983; 36: 731–6.
10 Bowling A. Choice of health indicator – the problem of measuring outcome. *Complementary Medical Research* 1988; 2(3): 43–63.

11 Higginson I, ed. *Clinical audit in palliative care*. Oxford: Radcliffe Medical Press, 1993.
12 Higginson I, McCarthy M. Validity of the support team Assessment Schedule: views of patients and families. *Palliative Medicine* 1993; 7: 219–28.
13 Higginson I, McCarthy M. Validity of a measure of palliative care – comparison with a quality of life index. *Palliative Medicine* 1994; 8 (4): 282–90.
14 Evans C, McCarthy M. Prognostic uncertainty in terminal care: can the Karnofsky index help? *Lancet* 1985; i: 1204–6.
15 Higginson I, Wade A, McCarthy M. Effectiveness of two palliative care support teams. *J Public Health Med* 1992; 14 (1): 50-6.
16 McCarthy M, Higginson I. Clinical audit by a palliative care team. *Palliative Medicine* 1991; 5 (3): 215–21.
17 McDaid P. STAS items for hospice day care. *STAS Users Newsletter* 1994; 1: 6–7.
18 Ramsay M. *A project to identify outcome measures for community services for people with dementia*. London: Faculty of Public Health Medicine, 1994.
19 Ramsay M, Winget C, Higginson I. A review of measures to determine the outcome of community services for people with dementia. *Age and Ageing* (in press).

4 Whose outcome is it anyway?

MARIANNE RIGGE

I will consider how information, or the lack of it, and good communication, or the lack of it, can affect patient choice and as a direct or indirect result of this, how outcomes may also be affected.

The first hat I wear (in the purely metaphorical sense) is director of the College of Health, a charity which aims to give people the information they need to help them make the most effective use of the health service; it also aims to improve the quality and quantity of communication between health service professionals and the patients they serve. We have done this in a variety of ways over the past 10 years. For example, we pioneered the provision of information to patients about hospital waiting lists with the publication of a series of annual guides from 1984 to 1991. Previously, there had been no accessible published information to alert the public to the fact that there was, and indeed remains, an astonishing variation in the length of time people have to wait for admission to hospital for operations. In the process we learnt a great deal about inequality of access and how much this can affect the quality of people's lives as well as their livelihoods and, ultimately, the quality of the outcome of treatment once they do receive it. Over the years we have had countless letters of thanks from people who felt that they or their relatives might have died had it not been for the information they were able to get about where they could ask their general practitioner to refer them for earlier treatment.

Since 1991, thanks to grants from the NHS Management

Executive, we have been able to help over 20 000 people in a much more direct way, through the National Waiting List Helpline. This incorporates the only computerised national database on waiting times for outpatient and inpatient waiting lists, not just by specialty but now also by consultant. Sadly, the NHS Executive no longer has a Waiting Times Initiative Fund and there is a real danger that the National Waiting List Helpline may have to close. We are in fact urgently seeking an alternative source of funding because we would like to develop the helpline into a centre for information about where to go for specialist treatment.

Providing health information over the telephone

Over the years the College of Health has also pioneered the provision of health information on a wide range of health and medical subjects by means of tapes which can be listened to over the telephone in complete confidentiality and anonymity in a service we call Healthline. Originally launched in 1984 with charitable funding, the service was free apart from the cost of an ordinary telephone call, but had to be discontinued in 1989 when lack of funding and competition from premium rate services running on 0898 numbers forced us out of business. Happily, the wheel has turned: with the advent of the single national freephone number and network of Regional Health Information Services, we were asked by North East Thames to run the service for that region when it was set up in 1992 and we were able to incorporate the Healthline tapes into this. On weekdays, callers get through to an operator who can give them information about the complete range of health services, self help groups, voluntary organisations, etc, throughout the region, as well as playing them tapes if they would find it helpful.

Now, thanks to a grant from the Department of Health which has enabled us to computerise the tapes, anyone living in North East Thames with access to a pushbutton telephone can listen to any of our 370 tapes at night and at the weekends. The subjects include common health problems which people can deal with themselves as well as illnesses for which they will need to consult a general practitioner or hospital doctor. They explain the signs and symptoms, the likely treatments, their alternatives and risks, and, importantly, what people can do to help themselves. We hope shortly to offer the service to all the other regional health information services so that, in theory, anyone in England could have access to consumer-friendly information on medical and health topics 24 hours a day.

Consumer audit

Another important area of the College of Health's work which has been developed over the past six years or so is what we call consumer audit – the application of a range of qualitative research methods such as observation; in depth, semistructured interviews; and focus group discussions to find out what patients, their carers, and potential users of health services think about them and want from them. We have worked for purchasers and providers across the range of acute, community, and primary care and, more recently, with social service departments. In the 30 or more consumer audit studies we have so far carried out, we have never yet failed to come up with findings that surprised the clinicians and managers who commissioned our research and led to immediate changes in practice. These did not necessarily cost a lot of money to implement since they often involved improvements in the quality of communication and information rather than expensive new fabric or equipment. And we have learnt that the people best placed to tell you about those key elements of clinical audit – access, process, and outcome – are the patients themselves.

My work at the College of Health has given me an insight into the wide ranging problems that consumers have in their everyday dealings with the health service. It has also enabled me to see how and why so many people are so deeply appreciative of the care they receive.

I am also one of the two lay members of the Clinical Outcomes Group whose work Calman has discussed in chapter 1. At the group's meetings I have learnt that there is a very real commitment to securing the involvement of consumers in clinical audit and outcomes. I have been impressed by the plethora of initiatives aimed at improving our knowledge of clinical effectiveness and outcomes.

Problems with league tables

What are the problems from the point of view of consumer organisations like mine which try to give patients information about how to make the most effective use of the NHS?

Publishing league tables is quite the fashion nowadays, but it is rather a hazardous one in the absence of rigorous definitions of what it is you are measuring. Take the one in the Patient's Charter about being immediately assessed when a patient gets to the accident and emergency department of the local hospital. This "immediate assessment" can consist of a process called "eyeballing" – after which the patient may wait four hours or more to get treated, even if the hospital comes out top of the league. Not very helpful from the patient's point of view.

However, doctors have their problems with league tables too, as we learnt when we published the Guide to Hospital Waiting Lists. Patients may have written to us expressing their profound gratitude, but so did surgeons expressing their strongest objections. Often these were that the information – supplied by their own health authorities – was inaccurate or out of date. That certainly seems to be a continuing problem. But many complained that their waiting lists were only as long as they are because they are known to be good surgeons, and they asked how their patients were to know whether a surgeon with a suspiciously short waiting list was any good at all. That is a good question and it's one which patients might well ask too.

Successive reports from CEPOD (now the National Confidential Enquiry into Peri-Operative Deaths) and many of the other reports beginning to emerge about effectiveness and outcomes, not to mention pretty well any edition of the specialist medical journals, have identified variations in medical practice that are sometimes unacceptable. Unfortunately, however, none of the published reports, whether or not financed by the taxpayer, enable identification of the hospital or doctor with unacceptably high rates of complications or the poorest outcomes.

Some of the reasons for this are understandable and they include the need for much better education of the public so that, for example, they understand that the surgeon with the highest mortality rate may be the one who is prepared to take on the worst cases. My own view is that the best possible way to achieve public understanding of such matters would be to go ahead and publish information about mortality and morbidity with proper explanations of the reasons for variations which may be entirely valid and thereby encourage informed public debate.

Identifying centres of expertise

In the absence of this, however, there is another problem which consumer organisations face when we are trying to help patients. If you cannot identify doctors you would rather not be referred to, the obvious solution is to turn the problem round and ask whether you can find out where the centres of expertise and best practice are. The minute you start trying to do this, however, all the rhetoric of informed choice starts to crumble away.

The public are nowadays bombarded with information about advances in medical treatment with new technology and drugs, minimally invasive surgery techniques, and so on, and they are also beginning to be well informed about the importance of being treated by someone who has been properly trained in the new techniques or by a specialist. Recently there have been reports from respiratory medicine specialists that some patients are getting suboptimal care because of a shortage of consultants. I discovered not so long ago that in some districts there are no cardiologists, though I have yet to hear of a district where there are no patients with coronary heart disease.

The problem is that there is no systematic way to get reliable, up to date information about centres of expertise, or about consultants who specialise within their specialty. Not only does this fly in the face of all the talk about informed choice in the Patient's Charter but it is compounded by the fact that, under the new systems of contracting, even well informed patients may find that there is no possibility of being treated by the consultant of their choice because money for extracontractual referrals is in short supply or the criteria for allowing them are restrictive. If patients want to find out about particular specialists, the stock answer from any of the medical institutions, be it the royal colleges, the BMA, or the General Medical Council, is that their general practitioner will know where to refer them. But that simply is not true in many cases. Where are the general practitioners supposed to get the information from?

Our health information service recently had an inquiry from a patient who had heard that trials were about to start in this country of a promising new drug for multiple sclerosis. As someone badly affected by the disease, she not unnaturally wanted to know how she might get involved in the trial. Her general practitioner had no idea so she got in touch with us. Our detective work started with the Multiple Sclerosis Society, who were helpful and gave us the name of the company that makes the drug concerned. Their information division was also helpful, up to a point. They told me that trials were about to start in 10 centres around the country. But when I asked if they could tell me where these were they said that they were not allowed to give out that information, but that the patient's general practitioner would know. Since I already knew that he didn't, I did some lateral thinking and decided that the National Hospital for Neurology and Neurosurgery would be a sensible starting point.

I have long since learnt that when ringing any hospital to find out about what services they provide, there is no point in asking for the information officer. If there is one, patient information is the last thing they are likely to deal with. The medical secretaries are a much better bet, and so it proved this time. The first one I spoke to didn't know about the trial involving multiple sclerosis patients but said she would ask her colleagues and ring me back. Ten minutes later I had a call to say that, yes, they were involved in the trial and that it was to start later in the summer; but there were already some 200 patients on the consultant's list who would like to be included and only 25 could be, of whom half would be given placebo. Having got this far, the least I could do was to find out who the consultant was, so that the woman who had got in touch with us could be referred to him by her general practitioner and stand a chance along with the others. The secretary said that she didn't think that she was allowed to tell me but that she was sure the patient's general practitioner would know. It didn't seem fair to ask her how the general practitioner would know, since she had been so helpful and it was by now clear that it is received wisdom that general practitioners know these things, perhaps by some form of osmosis. As it turned out, she relented and told me the consultant's name, which I duly passed on to the patient. Of course, it's extremely unlikely that she will get into the trial, but at least she has had the chance to take an informed part in her own health care and it is just possible that she will feel better for it.

Importance of communication

That brings me onto the second cause for concern in the question of consumer involvement in outcomes. Our consumer audit studies over the years have shown time and again the importance of the quality of communication between health professionals and their patients. Failures in communication can lead to poor uptake of services, poor compliance with treatment, feelings of disempowerment and helplessness, and, as a more or less direct result of all these, poor outcomes. The box gives an example – it is an extract from one of the case studies in a consumer audit we carried out on mental health services for elderly people.

In talking about outcomes, it is all too easy to concentrate on the sort that are easiest to measure, such as uncomplicated recovery from surgery. But for many people, especially those with long term chronic or incurable illness, a successful outcome may be impossible unless it is defined as keeping symptoms under

---

Mrs B is a 79 year old widow whose husband died in 1986. She lives alone in an isolated rural environment. After the death of her husband, Mrs B had approached her GP for help and support as she felt unable to live without her husband. After three visits, the GP told her she had no reason to worry and that she should stop bothering him. There was no further contact with the GP for a period of three years.

In November 1989 Mrs B's GP did refer her to a psychiatrist as she was still suffering from depression, and she was given several courses of antidepressants. Unfortunately she reacted badly to the medication and became suicidal, so she was allocated a community psychiatric nurse.

She greatly appreciated this and relied heavily on the visits of the nurse to keep her going through her loneliness. And she was also grateful that the nurse arranged for her to change to a new GP, not least because she had developed problems of pain around her neck and down the side of her legs. At the time of the interview, however, she had been given a general appointment to see the new GP in two months' time and she said that she didn't feel able to ask for an appointment before then for the new problems, because the GP might get angry with her. Her previous poor experience had taken away any confidence she might have had that the new doctor would take her seriously.

control and above all being made to feel in control. Here again the importance of good information and communication cannot be underestimated.

I would like to illustrate the point in the words of three patients talking about the help they received, not from health professionals, but from voluntary organisations, the Stroke Association and an incontinence support group. "They sent me home from hospital with no information, no help, and nowhere to turn to. I was so confused; I thought, is this it, then? I wished I'd died. I learnt more from you in half an hour than I did in three weeks from the hospital staff."

The second patient, also a stroke sufferer said, "Until now, I thought I was uniquely abnormal, because grown men don't cry."

And the third, a woman: "Thank God I heard about you. I've always been incontinent but I just couldn't find out where to get help. The local chemist said all I had to do was go to the GP. The GP said, no, the district nurse is for that. She said, no, you need social services; and the social worker told me I should see my own GP."

By contrast, when things work well, it is almost always because a professional has taken the time and trouble to communicate effectively. This is how a woman with breast cancer described her experience of hearing the bad news. "I can't speak highly enough of the doctor. He was very gentle and kind and didn't hurry even though it was a busy clinic. He let me get dressed, then he sat me down and asked what I thought was wrong. When I said 'cancer' he said that was right but I shouldn't worry too much as the lump was small. When he'd let that sink in a bit, he asked me if I knew about all the different treatments and the pros and cons. He asked me if I'd understood and whether I had anyone outside to take me home or if there was anyone the nurse could phone for me. He told me there was no hurry and that he wanted me to go home and think about what treatment I wanted and come back next week to talk again. He gave me the number of a nurse counsellor and asked me to get in touch with her if I was worried or I hadn't understood. It might seem funny, but I went out feeling really comforted and confident."[1]

I put that quote from one of our consumer audits into the booklet on breast cancer which was published as part of the Secretary of State's Patient Perception initiative – it was a pretty good outcome for the consultant as well as for the patient. Some aspects of the quality of care can be judged by one person alone, the person on the receiving end.

1 NHS Management Executive. *Breast Cancer*. London: Department of Health, 1993.

5 Outcomes in mental health

JOHN SHANKS

Why do outcomes seem so difficult?

To the busy clinician, the prospect of measuring outcomes is apt to elicit emotions of apathy and dismay. To the psychiatrist, any emotional state should prompt the question, "Why?" It may be worth examining why outcomes can seem at once challenging and profoundly uninteresting. The sense of difficulty comes from the perception of outcome measurement as being the province of research. This may be because a special, vaguely technical word like "outcome" implies that measurement will require a special technical instrument such as a health rating scale or standardised questionnaire. These instruments are the product of research and were often designed with research, rather than routine clinical practice, in mind. The multicentre, multi million dollar US Medical Outcomes Study is worlds away from the scarce resources of a busy NHS day hospital or outpatient clinic. Understandable, then, to feel that incorporating outcome measurement into day to day clinical practice would require the practice to become rather more like research. Since this is unlikely and probably undesirable, it comes to seem unlikely and probably undesirable that outcome measurement would ever find its way into normal practice.

Outcome = result

I propose that, far from being basically a research activity,

49

outcomes are a fundamental part of traditional clinical practice and that all experienced clinicians already know a great deal about outcomes. I also propose, perhaps recklessly, that measuring outcomes is easy. This is because outcomes are basically results by a different name. Both clinicians and patients have always been keenly interested in results, and both always attempt to assess results. Even the radical next step of payment by results is nothing new – physicians in ancient China were remunerated only so long as the patient remained well, an incentive towards effective practice which would probably render unnecessary the contemporary audit and clinical guidelines movement.

Rather than starting with research based classifications or instruments, I propose to look first for suitable outcome measures within traditional clinical practice and to resort to research only for supplementation or clarification.

Points of view

What results are the service user and the clinical team looking for, and what difference might it make to their interaction if these results were measured more systematically than at present? From the user's perspective, the desired result always differs, depending on which user we consider. Nowhere does it differ more dramatically than in mental health services. A good result from the patient's point of view may be a somewhat chaotic and precarious independence in the community. The patient's overburdened family may view this same result with apprehension as a poor alternative to residential care. An alarmed local community which perceives mentally ill people as violent criminals might prefer that care be provided from a base which is not only residential but locked. Referral agents, such as general practitioners, have a point of view on what they want from a mental health service, and this may be different again.

The clinical team is likely to give precedence to improvement in the clinical status of the patient – in symptoms, clinical signs, behaviour in the clinical setting. Although we sometimes feel as mental health practitioners that we are uniquely challenged by the highly unusual perspective of some of our patients, in fact we share with most other areas of health the problem that the patient's point of view often differs from that of the clinician, the carer, or the rest of society. The problem of what weighting to give to each of the competing viewpoints may require a service to define who is the prime client. This may not be the patient, but the carers or the community who seek treatment on behalf of a troubling or troublesome individual. A psychotherapy service all of whose patients are voluntary clients must adopt a different balance of perspectives in measuring outcomes than a forensic psychiatry service whose patients are invariably dangerous and usually detained under the Mental Health Act for the protection of others.

Identifying results to measure

What sorts of results then are both feasible to measure and deserving of the description "outcome?" Some examples are suggested in box 1. Of these types, only rating scales are in any way specialised. Different types of outcome will suit different circumstances: measurement of the frequency and severity of relapse would be particularly relevant to a service for chronic relapsing conditions such as schizophrenia, depression or alcohol misuse. A service for homeless people with mental illness might

---

Box 1 – Results that can be called outcomes

Traditional clinical assessment

Sentinel events
>   Relapse
>   Suicide
>   Violent incidents

Functional status markers
>   Employment
>   Accommodation

Satisfaction with care

Rating scales
>   Global Assessment Scale
>   Beck Depression Inventory
>   Other scales

---

select as a main outcome measure its success rate in placing clients in secure accommodation. Most mental health services will face an increased risk of suicide among their clients and so this sentinel event will regularly form part of a portfolio of outcomes.

The proposal to use suicide rate as an outcome measure is the example which often illustrates most clearly one of the real difficulties about outcomes – attribution. To what extent is suicide (or come to that, any of the other measures mentioned) under the control of a health service or any other service? Is not suicide, like mental health generally, more a product of social and personal circumstances than of treatment?

This dilemma may be expressed epigrammatically:

The problem with process measures is contributional validity
The problem with outcome measures is attributional validity

In other words, we may wonder what contribution an observed process, such as treatment, makes to the final result. We may equally wonder to what cause we should attribute an observed outcome.

Interpreting results

Measuring outcomes is fairly easy, but interpreting the results, once measured, may be more complex. We may find that we are able to measure subjective wellbeing with quite high levels of reliability and validity only to discover that it is uncertain to what extent any change in wellbeing is the result of treatment as opposed to external factors. Is there any point in measuring such health outcomes if they are unattributable? I suggest that there is; it is worthwhile knowing accurately how someone is and how they are progressing, even if we cannot say precisely why.[1] If results are to be used to compare services or to hold them to account, then it becomes necessary to disentangle the effect of service intervention from those extraneous factors such as social circumstances or life events. It becomes necessary to move from measures which are health outcomes to those which are health care outcomes, attributable to service interventions.

A question of attribution

How are we to know if the treatment we administered caused

the changes we observe or which patients perceive? Box 2 shows some possibilities.

Mental health practitioners are acutely aware of the limitations of the randomised controlled trial and the numerous areas of practice which do not fit easily into this powerful but demanding design. It may be particularly important therefore to explore alternative means of casting light on what cause is responsible for an observed effect. The accumulation of observations associating a particular treatment or intervention with a particular type of good or bad result is one such way of approaching this issue. Clinical audit may be an appropriate means of doing this. Associations can then be tested by established scientific rules of evidence[2] to assess the likelihood that there is a causal link between a particular intervention and the result which is observed to follow. Sometimes audit will indicate an area of practice where results seem strikingly good or bad and which would therefore be fruitful territory for more formal investigation by research.[3]

Not by outcomes alone

There could be a tendency to regard measures of the process and structure of treatment as poor substitutes for outcome. The need to record associations between process and outcome in order to accumulate evidence on cause and effect is one good reason for continuing to collect process information alongside outcomes.

Even where we can measure an outcome, we may sometimes

Box 2 – Attributing changes to treatment

Research
> Randomised controlled trials
> Meta-analysis

Audit
> Indicate areas for research

Cross design synthesis
> Test for causal links in associations of observed process and outcome

quite appropriately choose a proxy measure of process instead. Provided we have first established the connection between them, this is quite acceptable. We may know, for example, that maintaining serum lithium levels within a certain stated range reliably reduces the frequency and severity of relapse in certain types of manic-depressive psychosis. If so, then a service for people with manic-depressive psychosis might quite appropriately select as an outcome measure the serum lithium levels achieved by patients on treatment, since this is a proxy for the reduction in risk of relapse into psychosis. It is much more convenient to measure and represent serum lithium levels than to assess levels of depression or mania.

Standards of comparison

Deciding whether a particular outcome is good or bad requires some standard of comparison. Since initial severity of illness is one of the strongest predictors of final outcome, it is usually necessary to have some measure of how well or ill people are at the point of entry. Unfortunately, a simple before and after comparison will not always suffice. Deterioration over time may represent a therapeutic triumph if it involves slowing down the inevitable decline of a progressive disorder such as dementia. Equally, an improvement over time may be a poor outcome if it is less than that which would have occurred naturally without treatment.

The most satisfactory baseline for comparison would be the unmodified clinical course of the untreated condition. We should at least do better than that with treatment. But, especially for the more severe mental illnesses, it would be difficult and unethical to observe patients untreated for comparison purposes. We may be able to derive some information from historical records before effective treatments were available. Or we may find useful data in published research of the results obtained in other services. There is a growing industry in meta-analysis, combining the results of many different research trials of treatment to provide more precise estimates of result than could be derived from any one trial alone.[4] If no suitable published research is available then it may be necessary to establish a local baseline by simply observing for a time the progress of current service users and then taking this as the standard against which to judge future improvements.

Rating scales and questionnaires

The use of rating scales and standardised questionnaires introduces an additional level of complexity to outcome measurement but one which may sometimes be justified by the increased precision or detail they can provide. A wide range of rating scales for measuring both physical and mental health is available.[5, 6] Many were designed for use in research settings and are too lengthy or demanding for use in routine clinical practice, but there are brief and simple scales which can be used in normal clinical practice.[7]

A trade off must often be made between breadth and depth of coverage and between comprehensiveness and feasibility in use.

Self completion scales are attractive because they tap into subjective perceptions and because patients and carers often spend time waiting around in services, and this time can be utilised to fill in a scale or complete a form for subsequent analysis of progress.

Results matter

For all their problems, outcome measures have one great advantage. In scientific language, they have self evident validity. To put it plainly, results matter. It is worth taking some trouble to improve the way in which we measure them so that they can better inform the difficult decisions which both patients and clinicians must make.

1 Shanks JFA, Frater A. Health status outcomes and attributability. Is a red rose red in the dark? *Quality in Health Care* 1993; 2: 259–62.
2 Hill AB. The environment and disease. Association and causation. *Proc R Soc Med* 1965; 58: 295–300.
3 Smith R. Audit and research. *BMJ* 1992; 305: 905–6.
4 Piccinelli M, Wilkinson G. Outcome of depression in psychiatric settings. *Br J Psychiatry* 1994; 164: 297–304.
5 Thompson C, ed. *The instruments of psychiatric research.* Chichester: Wiley, 1989.
6 McDowell I, Newell C. *Measuring health. A guide to rating scales and questionnaires.* Oxford: Oxford University Press, 1987.
7 Endicott J, Spitzer RL, Fliess JL, Cohen J. The Global Assessment Scale, a procedure for measuring the overall severity of psychiatric disturbance. *Arch Gen Psychiatry* 1976; 33: 766–71.

6 Using outcome information to improve acute care: total hip replacement surgery

MARK WILLIAMS

Elective total hip replacement surgery is performed primarily to relieve the discomfort (pain and stiffness) and disability caused by arthropathies of the hip, particularly osteoarthritis.[1] Total hip replacement has been widely practised in the United Kingdom for over 25 years, and many people have now had this operation.[1, 2]

The considerable controversy that has surrounded the unmet demand for total hip replacement surgery, as reflected by long waiting lists, has tended to obscure the important issue, that the outcomes of primary surgery, in terms of technical success, morbidity and patient satisfaction, are very variable.[3] This has led to concern that the proportion of operations accounted for by costly and technically demanding revision procedures may increase to 30% or more, depending on the success of primary hip replacement.[4] In addition, there has been a demand for audit data on the failure rates of total hip replacement in orthopaedic units.[1]

The importance of evaluating the results of total hip replacement has been widely recognised for many years.[5–9] However, outcome assessment has been hampered by a lack of standardised terminology, missing or non-quantifiable clinical information, small samples, short periods of follow up, and emphasis on physicians' definitions of relief of pain and on measures of technical success rather than on patients' satisfaction or quality of life.[1–5, 7–9] The correlations between pain and motion of joints, functional independence, and psychological wellbeing are weak and inconsistent.[10, 11]

One of the current controversies surrounding total hip replacement surgery is the necessary outcome measures to be used. In addition, the evidence regarding the effectiveness and cost effectiveness of hip prostheses, and thromboprophylactic measures to prevent deep venous thrombosis and pulmonary embolism, are topics of considerable interest to purchasers of health care.

Outcome measures in total hip replacement surgery

In 1947 Gade described the prevailing disadvantages of outcome measures in orthopaedic surgery (box).[13] Since the 1940s several grading systems have been developed to rate the results of total hip replacement,[13–27] and the proliferation of such scales, without common descriptors or standard nomenclature, has made comparison of the findings of different investigators very difficult.[5]

The principal components of fifteen scales are summarised in table 6.1. Although most include measures of pain, joint geometry, and joint function, few include the patient's or the observer's perceptions and none consider social or emotional functioning. These instruments have, with few exceptions, not been tested for validity, reliability, or sensitivity. In recognition of these deficits the British Orthopaedic Association and the American Academy of Orthopedic Surgeons have attempted to

---

Outcome measures in orthopaedic surgery

"Too frequently one is obliged to accept the clinician's subjective and verbally expressed characteristics concerning the therapeutic results. As a rule these are expressed in terms such as: 'Very good,' 'Fairly good,' etc. Such terms make it very difficult to perform a comparative evaluation of different methods."

H G Gade (1947)[13]

Table 6.1 – Clinimetric properties of hip rating scales

Index	Year	Principal components								Reliability	Validity		
		1	2	3	4	5	6	7	8		F value	Correlation coefficient	Responsiveness
Gade	1947	+	+	-	-	-	-	-	-	-	+	-	-
Judet	1952	+	+	+	-	-	-	-	-	-	+	-	-
D'Aubigne	1954	+	+	+	-	-	-	-	-	-	+	-	-
Shepherd	1954	+	+	+	-	+	-	-	-	-	+	-	-
Stinchfield	1957	+	+	+	+	-	-	-	-	-	+	-	-
Larson	1963	+	+	+	+	-	-	-	-	-	+	-	-
Lazansky	1967	+	+	+	-	-	-	-	-	-	+	-	-
Harris	1969	+	+	+	-	-	-	-	-	-	+	-	-
Anderson	1972	+	+	+	-	-	-	-	-	-	+	+	-
Charnley	1972	+	+	+	-	-	-	-	-	-	+	-	-
HEF	1975	+	+	+	-	-	-	-	-	+	+	-	-
JOAHSM	1983	+	+	+	-	-	-	-	-	-	+	-	-
UCLA	1984	+	-	+	-	-	-	-	-	-	+	-	-
MHS	1985	+	-	+	-	-	-	-	-	-	+	+	-
Lequesne	1985	+	-	+	-	-	-	-	-	-	+	-	-

HEF = Hip Evaluation Form; JOAHSM = Japanese Orthopaedic Association Hip SCore Method; UCLA = University of California at Los Angeles; MHS = Mayo Hip Score.
1 = Pain, 2 = Joint geometry, 3 = Function, 4 = Muscle power, 5 = Global assessment (patients), 6 = Global assessment (observer), 7 = Social function, 8 = Emotional function.

improve and standardise the systems.[5, 12] Nevertheless, focus on patients' perceptions and quality of life has been lacking.[1] In addition, the interpretation of outcome studies must consider those variables that influence outcome.

Factors affecting outcome of total hip replacement

The factors which affect the success of total hip replacement include those related to the patient, such as diagnosis and general health, to the surgeon, including the operative technique, and to the institution in which the operation is done. These covariates distinguish between the results of the operation and the variables that might explain differences between individual surgeons or institutions. To ensure accuracy and reliability, considerable analytical capability and resources are needed for the collection and analysis of data on these items. Studies of operative results must account for factors critical to operative risk and outcome and control for them in statistical analyses.

Characteristics of patients

Age is important in terms of a patient's general health, functional goals, satisfaction and functional needs.[9]

Poverty is associated with a worse outcome for many surgical treatments.[28–30] Low socioeconomic status may affect access to health care, recognition that care is needed, communication with health care professionals, nutrition, housing conditions, etc.[31, 32]

Social support refers to resources in the environment that meet a person's needs. Studies on social support for patients who had rheumatic disease showed that it had a positive effect on the patient's functions.[33]

Primary diagnosis may affect risk and outcome. The underlying disease correlates, in part, with a risk of development of complications. The risk in a patient who has longstanding rheumatoid arthritis differs from that for a relatively healthy person in whom only one hip is affected. In addition, drugs used to treat the underlying disorder may influence the outcome. For example, steroids used to treat rheumatoid arthritis may increase the risk of infection and affect the patient's general health and employment status.

Factors affecting outcome of total hip replacement

Patients' characteristics:
 Age
 Poverty
 Social support
 Primary diagnosis

Indications for operation

Operative factors:
 Surgeon
 Operative techniques
 Type of prosthetic implant

Institutional characteristics:
 Volume of operations
 Rehabilitation staff
 Measures to counter postoperative infection

Medical condition:
 Comorbidity
 Health status
 Quality of life
 Risk of infection
 Drugs used by patient

Indications for operation

Indications for total hip replacement usually include refractory pain and disabling limitation of function. Which of the indications is more dominant may affect the success of the operation and the patient's expectations. The patient's decision to have the operation is sometimes determined by highly personal preferences or goals.[5]

Operative factors

The surgeon's experience, training and specialisation in total hip replacement are thought to have an important effect on the results of the operation.[5] The technical aspects of total hip replacement operations differ. Variations include the type of prosthesis, the operative exposure used and the adequacy of the bone stock.

60

Institutional characteristics

The characteristics of the hospital influence the results of an operation and correlate with some characteristics of the surgeon. The volume of operations performed in the institution is a strong determinant of mortality from total hip replacement and it is likely that volume also correlates with differences in surgical results and complications.[34] The relation between volume and outcome is not entirely clear because centres with large volumes may have different case mixes of patients. The availability of skilled rehabilitation staff might also affect the functional results and how long the patients stay in hospital.[35] In addition, features such as laminar air flow and isolator systems may reduce the rate of postoperative infections.[36, 37]

Medical condition

Concurrent active medical or operative problems may be associated with pain or loss of function, potentially confounding the outcome of total hip replacement.[38] Several instruments are available for quantifying comorbid conditions.[39] Measures of case mix for patients which were designed to predict mortality or the use of resources are less appropriate for studies of the results of elective total hip replacement.[40, 41]

In outcome studies a person's general health can be viewed as the outcome of the operation or as a covariate which may affect surgical results. Instruments have been developed for evaluating patients' general health and their health related quality of life, covering domains such as physical, social, and role function; symptoms; emotional status; cognition; and perception of one's health. These measures are particularly important in the evaluation of patients with chronic disease, for whom life expectancy is not greatly decreased and the quality of life is more relevant. The outcome of total hip replacement may be estimated by use of intervention specific measures and by generic measures. Figure 6.1 summarises the interrelation of these measures and the underlying disorders. Generic instruments permit comparisons across different types of interventions and diagnostic conditions, and intervention specific measures may be used for focusing on particular functional areas as they are more responsive to interventions specific to the disease. Recently investigators have attempted to increase the usefulness of these

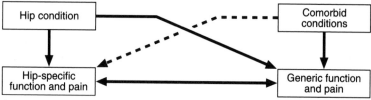

Figure 6.1 Model of associations among conditions specific and generic measures

measures by developing short instruments, and the relative ability of these instruments to discriminate change in clinical status is currently being researched.[42-47]

Risk factors for postoperative infection include previous surgery, rheumatoid arthritis, poor nutrition, steroid therapy, diabetes mellitus, and sites of pre-existing infection, including the urinary tract.[48-50]

An accurate list of drugs used by the patient provides important baseline data which relate to the severity and activity of the underlying disease. Drugs may also predispose to an increased rate of complications after total hip replacement. Steroids increase the fragility of the skin, predispose to infection, and impair healing of the wound.[51]

The dimensions of outcome assessment in total hip replacement surgery

Relief from the pain of an arthritic hip is one of the principal reasons for surgery and is a key component of the health status of a patient who has arthritis.[52] Pain can be measured with a variety

---

Dimensions of outcome assessment for total hip replacement

Pain
Occupational status
Activities of daily living
Gait
Physical examination
Patient's satisfaction and expectation
Complications

---

of techniques and, for patients who have musculoskeletal diseases, pain related function may be a more reliable method of assessment.[5] Various measures have been used including numerical scales and visual analogue scales. Since many patients who have a total hip replacement have discomfort from other joints, pain scales have also been linked to these specific joints. Analgesics or other drugs and the use of mobility aids affect the level of pain and should be considered in interpreting the patient's responses.[5]

For patients of working age, occupational status is important for stratification before surgery as it may relate to the severity of disease or the motivation of the patient. It is also a critical outcome of the operation, reflecting both improved function and increased economic productivity.[5]

The patient needs assessment of a number of activities of daily living related to the function of the hip and the ability to mobilise and make transfers, attend to personal hygiene, dress, etc.[5]

Gait is assessed according to whether assistive devices are needed and the distance that a patient can walk with or without such support should be measured.[5]

In a physical examination, the range of motion of the affected hip should be measured according to standardised criteria.[5]

Although objective measures of pain and function are critical parameters in the assessment of the results of total hip replacement, the goals and expectations of the patient, and the extent to which these are met by the operation, are also important. One study showed that expectations (satisfaction) regarding total hip replacement were met in only 55% of patients.[53] In another study, more than 90% of patients expressed satisfaction with total hip replacement; dissatisfaction was due primarily to persisting pain or poor walking capacity.[54] Patients' preferences with regard to particular symptoms are critical to the decision of whether or not to perform surgery. Measuring patients' expectations, preferences for particular clinical states, and satisfaction with the operation improves the selection of patients and provides a richer understanding of the outcome of total hip replacement.

Outcome assessment should evaluate both positive and negative aspects of the intervention, so that the net benefit to the patient can be estimated. Perioperative complications are defined as complications occurring during the operation and the two weeks after surgery. Complications must be assessed systematically, and to avoid observer bias the assessment should be performed by someone who is not involved with the operation.[5]

Published research on outcomes of total hip replacement

Outcome studies should ideally be performed prospectively, collecting information on a patient's status before and after surgery. A recent review of 648 published studies of 50 or more total hip replacement operations found that only 35 had collected data prospectively; the percentage of patients followed up varied between 19% and 100%, and the duration of follow up varied from less than one year to over 20 years.[55] Of the variables affecting outcome, the type of prosthesis was mentioned in 100% of studies but details regarding the surgeon were mentioned in only 8%. Information on other important variables influencing outcome included type of arthropathy (reported in 79% of studies), age (71%), socioeconomic status (2%), activities of daily living (10%), patients' expectations (1%), and social support (1%). The ability to interpret adverse outcomes has been compromised by this incomplete collection of potentially influential variables.

The lack of validity and reliability in measuring outcome has been described. A common measure of outcome in total hip replacement surgery, "survivorship," describes the longevity of the prosthetic implant.[56] The definition of survivorship varies, having been reported as the "need" for revision surgery (which includes both the surgeon's and the patient's preferences) and the radiologically defined survival of the prosthesis. Survivorship studies, which have mainly been conducted retrospectively, have also suffered from losses to follow up due to death, patient's refusal, or migration of patients. Small case series have resulted in increasingly wide confidence intervals constructed around the cumulative survival as the duration of follow up increases.[56]

Which hip prosthesis?

The lack of prospective randomised controlled trials, and the absence of statistical adjustment for the many variables that may influence outcome severely constrains conclusions regarding the most effective and cost effective hip implant. A recent study of prostheses used in 261 English hospitals found 30 different types of cemented prostheses and 35 uncemented prostheses in current use.[57] The Charnley low friction arthroplasty was used in 193 hospitals; in one English region it accounted for 62% of operations (unpublished data). The Charnley prostheses currently seem to have the best results in terms of longevity, with a failure rate of less than 1% a year.[58] It has been stated that any new prosthetic designs should be compared with the Charnley in a randomised controlled trial before they are adopted in clinical practice, but the logistics are formidable: to detect a 30% improvement in results for a new prosthesis, many thousands of patients would need follow up for a decade.[3]

The lack of quality assurance surrounding the introduction of new implants to the British market has been a source of concern. Controls in Britain do not compare with the stringent measures backed by legislation in France and the United States.[59]

Thromboprophylaxis in total hip replacement surgery

Stasis of the venous circulation in the leg, damage to the femoral vein during surgery, and change in the balance of coagulation factors have all been implicated in the development of deep venous thrombosis (DVT) and pulmonary embolus (PE) after total hip replacement surgery.[60] The incidence of DVT by venography after surgery has been estimated to be 40% or more.[60] The clinical incidence of DVT is 2% owing to the high proportion of subclinical cases and the acknowledged unreliability of clinical examinations.[61] Controversy still exists regarding the relative effectiveness of routine thromboprophylaxis as opposed to selective thromboprophylaxis in high risk cases. Recent research suggests that the death rate due to PE with selective thromboprophylaxis may be as low as 0.34% (95% confidence interval 0.09% to 0.88%), with the clinical incidence of PE being 1.2% (0.65% to 2.02%).[61]

Various prophylactic measures have been tried, including low molecular weight heparin, warfarin, antiplatelet agents (aspirin, for example), and pneumatic compression stockings. A meta-analysis of trials of prophylactic measures in major orthopaedic surgery showed a lower incidence of high risk proximal thrombosis and fatal PE when fixed dose heparin was used, but the overall number of thromboses was not reduced.[62] More recently, a meta-analysis of 13 trials of elective orthopaedic surgery by the Antiplatelet Trialists' Collaboration has found a reduction of DVT of 49% (SD 11%) and pulmonary embolism 51% (24%); absolute benefits for those receiving aspirin were higher in high risk patients.[63]

Thirty two different combinations of prophylactic measures were in use in the United Kingdom in 1992, with 25% of surgeons reporting no routine measure.[64] Further meta-analyses of existing evidence are in progress. Large scale trials of the various options in prophylaxis are still required, but the implications are again formidable: in order to detect a minimum reduction of death rate due to PE from 0.5% to 0.3%, 50 000 patients are required in a trial with 80% power and a significance level of 1%.

Future challenges in outcome measurement

Current published research on the outcomes of total hip replacement surgery consists primarily of clinician defined retrospective studies using unstandardised outcome measures, with the risk of selection and observer bias and lack of inclusion of patient perspectives. Research needs to take account of intervention specific measures that have been rigorously tested psychometrically and that include measures of patients' understanding, expectations, satisfaction, and quality of life. In addition, economic analyses will need to be incorporated in such studies.

Outcomes must be routinely recorded. Data has been collected from the national register of total hip replacements in Sweden since 1979. In the United Kingdom the Trent regional arthroplasty study, established in 1990, collects routine data at the time of total hip replacement surgery and follows patients up for 12 months. An aim of this large study, which has collected data on over 8000 total hip replacements to date, is to continue prospective follow up so as to evaluate long term outcomes using the multidimensional approach I have described.

1 Williams MH, Frankel SJ, Nanchahal K, Coast J, Donovan JL. Total hip replacement: epidemiologically based needs assessment. *In:* Stevens A, Raftery J, eds. *Health care needs Assessment*. Vol 1. Oxford: Radcliffe Medical Press, 1994: 448–523.
2 Williams MH, Newton JN, Frankel SJ, Braddon F, Barclay E, Gray JAM. Prevalence of

USING OUTCOME INFORMATION TO IMPROVE ACUTE CARE

total hip replacement: how much demand has been met? *J Epidemiol Community Health* 1994; **48**: 188–91.

3 Bulstrode CJK, Murray DW, Carr AJ, Pynsent PB, Carter SR. Designer hips. *BMJ* 1993; **306**: 732–3.
 4 Bulstrode CJK, Carr AJ, Murray DW. Prediction of future work-load in total joint replacement. *In:* Institution of Mechanical Engineers, Wallace WA, eds. *Joint replacement in the 1990s. Clinical studies, financial implications and marketing approaches.* Bury St Edmunds: Mechanical Engineering Publications, 1992: 25–7.
 5 Liang MH, Katz, JN, Phillips C, Sledge C, Cats-Baril W. The total hip arthroplasty evaluation form of the American Academy of Orthopaedic Surgeons. *J Bone Joint Surg* 1991; **73A**: 639–46.
 6 Codman EA. *The shoulder.* Boston: [privately printed], 1934.
 7 Galante J. The need for a standardized system for evaluating results of total hip surgery. *J Bone Joint Surg* 1985; **67A**: 511–2.
 8 Gartland JJ. Orthopaedic clinical research. Deficiences in experimental design and determinations of outcome. *J Bone Joint Surg* 1988; **70A**: 1357–64.
 9 Gross M. A critique of the methodologies used in clinical studies of hip-joint arthroplasty published in the English-language orthopaedic literature. *J Bone Joint Surg* 1988; **70A**: 1364–71.
10 Visuri T, Honkanen R. The influence of total hip replacement on selected activities of daily living and on the use of domestic aid. *Scand J Rehab Med* 1978; **10**: 221–4.
11 Wilcock GK. Benefits of total hip replacement to older patients and the community. *BMJ* 1978; **ii**: 37–9.
12 Muller ME, Sledge C, Poss R, Schatzker JH, Engel C, Paterson D. Report of the SICOT presidential commission on documentation and evaluation. *Int Orthop* 1990; **14**: 221–9.
13 Gade HG. A contribution to the surgical treatment of osteoarthritis of the hip joint: a clinical study. III. Comments on the follow-up examination and the evaluation of the therapeutic results. *Acta Chirug Scand* 1947; **120**(suppl): 37–45.
14 Judet R, Judet J. Technique and results with the acrylic femoral head prosthesis. *J Bone Joint Surg* 1952; **34B**: 173–80.
15 D'Aubigne RM, Postel M. Functional results of hip arthroplasty with acrylic prosthesis. *J Bone Joint Surg* 1954; **36A**: 451–75.
16 Shepherd MM. Assessment of function after arthroplasty of the hip. *J Bone Joint Surg* 1954; **36B**: 354–63.
17 Stinchfield FE, Copperman B, Shea CE Jr. Replacement of the femoral head by Judet or Austin Moore prosthesis. *J Bone Joint Surg* 1951; **39A**: 1043–58.
18 Larson C. Rating scale for hip disabilities. *Clin Orthop Rel Res* 1963; **31**: 85–93.
19 Lazansky MG. A method for grading hips. *J Bone Joint Surg* 1967; **49B**: 644–51.
20 Harris WH. Traumatic arthritis of the hip after dislocation and acetabular fractures: treatment by mold arthroplasty – an end-result study using a new method of result evaluation. *J Bone Joint Surg* 1969; **51A**: 737–55.
21 Andersson G. Hip assessment: a comparison of nine different methods. *J Bone Joint Surg* 1972; **54B**: 621–5.
22 Charnley J. The long-term results of low-friction arthroplasty of the hip performed as a primary intervention. *J Bone Joint Surg* 1972; **54B**: 61–76.
23 Ritter MA, Alpern GD, Connolly G. The reliability of a hip evaluation form. *Orthopaedic Review* 1975; **4**: 25–30.
24 Itami Y, Akamatsu N, Tomita M, Nagasi M, Nakajima I. A clinical study of the results of cementless total hip replacement. *Arch Orthop Traum Surg* 1983; **102**: 1–10.
25 Amstutz HC, Thomas BJ, Jinnah R, Kim W, Grogan T, Yale C. Treatment of primary osteoarthritis of the hip. *J Bone Joint Surg* 1984; **66A**: 228–41.
26 Kavanagh BF, Fitzgerald RH Jr. Clinical and roentgenographic assessment of total hip arthroplasty – a new hip score. *Clin Orthop Rel Res* 1985; **193**: 133–40.
27 Lequesne M. European guidelines for clinical trials of new antirheumatic drugs. *Eular Bulletin* 1980; **9**(Suppl 6): 171–5.
28 Egbert LD, Rothman JL. Relation between the race and economic status of patients and who performs their surgery. *N Engl J Med* 1977; **297**: 90–1.
29 Otten MW Jr, Teutsch SM, Williamson DF, Marks JS. The effect of known risk factors on the excess mortality of black adults in the United States. *JAMA* 1990; **263**: 845–50.
30 Yergan J, Flood AB, Logerfo JP, Diehr P. Relationship between patient race and the intensity of hospital services. *Med Care* 1987; **25**: 592–603.

67

31 Pincus T, Callahan LF. Formal education as a marker for increased mortality and morbidity in rheumatoid arthritis. *J Chron Dis* 1985; **38**: 973–84.

32 Pincus T, Callahan LF, Burkhauser RV. Most chronic diseases are reported more frequently by individuals with fewer than 12 years of formal education in the age 18–64 United States population. *J Chron Dis* 1987; **40**: 865–74.

33 Kaplan GA, Delongis A. Psychological Factors influencing the course of arthritis: a prospective study. Paper read at the American Psychological Association, Anaheim, California, August 1983.

34 Luft HS, Bunker JP, Enthoven AC. Should operations be regionalized? The empirical relation between surgical volume and mortality. *N Engl J Med* 1979; **301**: 1364–9.

35 Liang MH, Cullen KE, Larson MG, Schwartz JA, Robb-Nicholson C, Fossel AH, Roberge N, Poss R. Effects of reducing physical therapy services on outcomes in total joint arthroplasty. *Med Care* 1987; **25**: 276–85.

36 Nelson JP, Glassburn AR Jr, Talbott RD, McElhinney JP. The effect of previous surgery, operating room environment, and preventive antibiotics on postoperative infection following total hip arthroplasty. *Clin Orthop* 1980; **147**: 167–9.

37 Poss R, Thornhill TS, Ewald FC, Thomas WH, Batte NJ, Sledge CB. Factors influencing the incidence and outcome of infection following total joint arthroplasty. *Clin Orthop* 1984; **182**: 117–26.

38 Greenfield S. The state of outcome research: are we on target? *N Engl J Med* 1989; **320**: 1142–3.

39 Linn BS, Linn MW, Gurel L. Cumulative illness rating scale. *J Am Geriat Soc* 1968; **16**: 622–6.

40 Charlson ME, Pompei P, Ales KL, MacKenzie CR. A new method of classifying prognostic comorbidity in longitudinal studies. Development and validation. *J Chron Dis* 1987; **40**: 373–83.

41 Knaus WA, Draper EA, Wagner DP, Zimmerman JE. APACHE II: a severity of disease classification system. *Crit Care Med* 1985; **13**: 818–29.

42 Jette AM, Davies AR, Cleary PD, Calkins DR, Rubenstein LV, Fink A, et al. The functional status questionnaire: reliability and validity when used in primary care. *J Gen Intern Med* 1986; **1**: 143–9.

43 Nelson E, Wasson J, Kirk J, Keller A, Clark D, Dietrich A, et al. Assessment of function in routine clinical practice: description of the COOP chart method and preliminary findings. *J Chron Dis* 1987; **40**(suppl 1): 55–63S.

44 Pincus T, Summey JA, Soraci SA Jr, Wallston KA, Hummon NP. Assessment of patient satisfaction in activities of daily living using a modified Stanford health assessment questionnaire. *Arthrit Rheum* 1983; **26**: 1346–53.

45 Stewart AL, Hays RD, Ware JE Jr. The MOS short-form general health survey. Reliability and validity in a patient population. *Med Care* 1988; **26**: 724–35.

46 Wallston KA, Brown GK, Stein MJ, Dobbins CJ. Comparing the short and long versions of the arthritis impact measurement scales. *J Rheumatol* 1989; **16**: 1105–9.

47 Ware JE Jr. The SF36: an improved MOS short form health survey. Unpublished data.

48 D'Ambrosia RD, Shoji H, Heater R. Secondary infection in total joint replacements by hematogenous spread. *J Bone Joint Surg* 1976; **58A**: 450–3.

49 Gristina AG, Kolkin J. Current concepts review. Total joint replacement and sepsis. *J Bone Joint Surg* 1983; **65A**: 128–34.

50 Jensen JE, Jensen TG, Smith TK, Johnston DA, Dudrick SJ. Nutrition in orthopaedic surgery. *J Bone Joint Surg* 1982; **64A**: 1263–72.

51 Perhala RS, Wilke WS, Clough JD, Segal AM. Local infectious complications following large joint replacement in rheumatoid arthritis patients treated with methotrexate versus those not treated with methotrexate. *Arthrit Rheum* 1991; **34**: 146–52.

52 Kazis LE, Meenan RF, Anderson JJ. Pain and rheumatic diseases. Investigation of a key health status component. *Arthrit Rheum* 1983; **26**: 1017–22.

53 Burton KE, Wright V, Richards J. Patients' expectations in relation to outcome of total hip replacement surgery. *Ann Rheumat Dis* 1979; **38**: 471–4.

54 Kay A, Davison B, Badley E, Wagstaff S. Hip arthroplasty: patient satisfaction. *Br J Rheumatol* 1983; **22**: 243–9.

55 Williams MH. Total hip replacement: evidence of effectiveness. *Effective Health Care Bulletin*. University of Leeds (in press).

56 Carr AJ, Morris RW, Murray DW, Pynsent PB. Survival analysis in joint replacement surgery. *J Bone Joint Surg* 1993; **73B**: 178–82.

57 Newman KJH. Total hip and knee replacements: a survey of 261 hospitals in England. *J R Soc Med* 1993; **86**: 527–9.

58 McCoy TH, Salvati EA, Ranawat CS, Wilson PD. A fifteen year follow-up study of one hundred Charnley low friction arthroplasties. *Orthop Clin North Am* 1988; **19**: 467–76.

59 Faro LMC, Huiskes R. Quality assurance of joint replacement. *Acta Orthop Scand* 1992: **63**(Suppl 250): 1–33.

60 Merli GJ. Deep venous thrombosis and pulmonary embolism prophylaxis in orthopaedic surgery. *Med Clin North Am* 1993; **77**: 397–411.

61 Warwick DJ, Williams MH, Bannister GC. Death and thromboembolic disease after total hip replacement, *Journal of Bone and Joint Surgery* (in press).

62 Collins R, Scrimgeour A, Yusuf S, *et al.* Reduction in fatal pulmonary embolism and venous thrombosis by peri-operative administration of subcutaneous heparin. *N Engl J Med* 1988; **318**: 1162–73.

63 Antiplatelet Trialists' Collaboration. Collaborative overview of randomised trials of antiplatelet therapy. III. *BMJ* 1994; **308**: 235–36.

64 Owen TD, Coorsh J. The use of thromboprophylaxis in total hip replacement surgery: are the attitudes of orthopaedic surgeons changing? *J Roy Soc Med* 1992; **85**: 679–81.

7 Auditing the outcome of total knee replacement

MARTIN BARDSLEY, ROBERT CLEARY

This chapter draws on experience at the Freeman Hospital in Newcastle upon Tyne, where the assessment of outcome as part of an audit process was developed in a number of conditions, one of which was knee replacement.[1] The work on knee replacement has subsequently been extended to cover a number of sites across what was the Northern Regional Health Authority.[2] This chapter outlines the way that outcome measures were developed in this setting and considers some of the problems encountered.

The context for monitoring outcome

Though improvement in patient outcome is often cited as a fundamental goal of the health service, our ability to measure those outcomes and to assess the value of inputs in terms of the health benefit they give is extremely limited. For knee replacements the concerns have traditionally been with the longevity of a prosthesis,[3] though there is an increasing interest in more sophisticated assessments.[4]

Though we can probably all agree that we need to improve our grasp of the outcomes of care, the way we choose and apply outcome measures depends on the context in which we are using them. For example, different outcome measures might be used in

70

clinical trials rather than for clinical audit of quality assurance for a purchasing health authority.

This study focused on the process of audit – namely, developing appropriate outcome measures that clinicians could use to inform the process of care. Though it originally started in one hospital, a streamlined data set has subsequently been applied to over 12 hospitals across one region and the results pooled for over 1400 patients.

Identifying outcome measures

The process of identifying and implementing outcome measurement within the study followed through three stages expected of any audit process: defining the objectives of care; selecting the methods for measurement; and monitoring outcome and examining departures from the agreed standard.

Defining objectives

The first step was to clarify with the clinical team what health improvement they were expecting to observe in patients receiving a knee replacement. This involved identifying:

- the key reference groups of patients and how they might be defined;
- the expected time for improvements to occur; and
- most important confounding variables, ones that were felt to be strongly linked to good or bad outcome.

Selecting methods for measurement

Choosing the appropriate ways to measure the outcome was an important stage and involved testing and piloting different approaches. The criteria used in selecting scales covered:

- construct validity – did it measure what we wanted it to measure?
- content validity – did the measure address those aspects of health relevant to these patients?
- using existing scales rather than inventing new ones;
- reliability;

71

- responsiveness – was the scale able to show change over time;[5] and
- practicality, balancing the cost of data collection with the validity and utility of that information.

Though this work sought to use routine data sources as much as possible, additional data have been collected from patients. There has been an investment in coordination through audit staff within the Freeman and in all sites contributing to the regional study.

Monitoring outcome

Systems for collecting data used a combination of patient and physician completed questionnaires (box). The original work at the Freeman collected more data than did the subsequent multihospital study. Postal follow ups were used; response rates when questionnaires were posted to patients were good (typically over 80%). Data were aggregated and reported back to the clinical team in reports and meetings; these included:

- comparisons of groups of patients;
- identification of pattern of individuals (typically those with poorer outcomes); and
- comparisons between hospitals.

Changes in outcome measures

Technical/clinical measures

Knee function scores have been widely used in the assessment of knee replacements,[6] and include the Knee Society Rating Scale, which assesses pain, technical issues such as stability, range of motion, alignment of the joint, and some assessment of function, such as walking distance and ability to climb stairs.[7] These different elements are scored by the clinician in the presence of the patient. The scale has the advantage of incorporating many elements of the clinical assessment of the patient into a structured format which can be integrated into a routine consultation. Repeated measurement enables changes in score to be observed.

Figure 7.1 illustrates the typical change in knee scores three months after operation. Significant improvements were observed

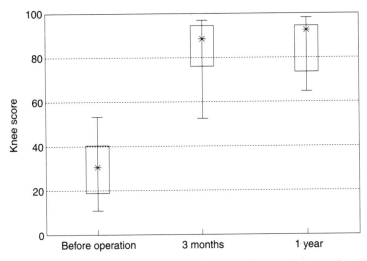

Figure 7.1 Changes in knee score 12 months after total knee replacement for 198 patients with osteoarthritis. Figure shows median scores (*), interquartile ranges (box), and 10th and 90th centiles (bars)

to three months, with little subsequent change to a year. As an outcome measure knee function score has the advantage of being relatively easy to use, understandable to clinicians, and potentially common to different centres and different studies. The disadvantages are that the scoring may be a little arbitrary; the score may not represent the full range of patient's lifestyle, and it could suffer from problems of inter-rater reliability.

Another outcome was concerned with loosening of the prosthesis as seen on radiographs. Once again, established scoring systems exist to assess the degree of loosening,[8] yet these take time to complete. The scoring system we tried aims to grade the thickness of radiolucent lines in 12 distinct zones – a cumbersome process compared with the clinician's visual check. In practice we found problems with completing these forms consistently. They were not subsequently used in the multi-hospital audit.

Several complications of treatment were also considered. In theory, important complications should be recorded in medical notes. The process of outcome assessment should structure that information more formally and enable aggregation across patient groups. The problems with this type of data are, firstly, that definitions can be difficult, especially across a number of different sites – what exactly do we mean by a wound infection? Secondly, the frequency with which the complications arise may be small; for example, one study of the frequency of deep venous thrombosis or pulmonary embolism found an incidence of 1.7% in 1909 patients undergoing knee arthroplasty.[9]

General health scales

There is an increasing recognition that the outcomes of care go beyond the traditional clinical view to encompass wider aspects of a person's health status and general wellbeing. A range of measurement instruments has been developed to assess general health across a number of dimensions, covering physical, psychological, and social function.[10, 11] Such scales typically exist as patient completed questionnaires where simple yes/no responses are elicited to a series of carefully designed questions. The structure of the best examples of these scales has been carefully developed and subjected to rigorous testing for validity and reliability.[12, 13]

Some scales are specific to a particular condition – for example, the Arthritis Impact Measurement Scales.[14] Others are generic instruments potentially applicable to a range of conditions, the most common being the Sickness Impact Profile,[15] Nottingham Health Profile,[16] and the ubiquitous SF-36.[17, 18]

This study chose the Nottingham Health Profile, a generic instrument with 38 questions covering six dimensions of health: pain, mobility, energy, social isolation, sleep, and emotional reactions. This was chosen as an example of a well tested generic scale where the dimensions were felt to be relevant to the patient group. It was also consistent with other studies used at the Freeman, which gave advantages in comparing scores between diverse categories, and familiarity with processing the data.

The key concern was with the ability of the scale to be responsive to clinical change in this patient group.[19, 20] Figure 7.2 shows the improvements in scores of the Nottingham Health Profile from admission to 3 months and one year after the operation for one subset of patients, women aged over 65. The changes in scores were significant on all dimensions but especially for energy, sleep, pain, and mobility. These observed changes lend validity to the scale. Once again the benefits of the procedure were manifest in the first three months, with less change to 12 months. Comparison with Nottingham Health Profile scores from

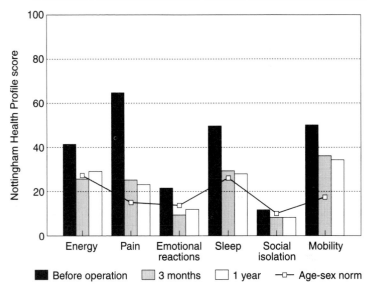

Figure 7.2 Mean Nottingham Health Profile scores to 12 months postoperatively for 100 women aged over 65 compared with age-sex norms

other samples suggested that postoperatively patients are in a poorer state of health than the age/sex norm, especially regarding pain and mobility, but are roughly comparable on the other dimensions.

The Nottingham Health Profile could also detect differences between hospitals. Figure 7.3 compares mean improvements in the pain dimensions across different hospitals.

Finally, it should be noted that there are other dimensions of outcome that may be important but were not considered in this work. One concerns patients' satisfaction with the process of care;[21] linked to this is an assessment of patients' expectations.[22]

Changing practice?

This study of outcomes of knee replacement has yielded some useful results concerning the ways we monitor outcome and the types of scale that can be used.

- Statistically significant improvements in knee score and Nottingham Health Profile score can be observed to 3 months after operation; subsequent change to 12 months is less.

75

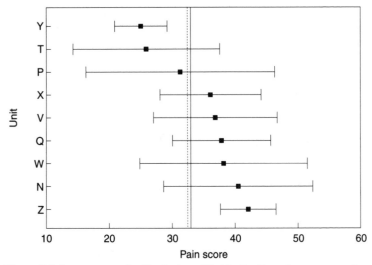

Figure 7.3 Improvement in Nottingham Health Profile pain scores to three months postoperatively for nine hospitals in Northern region (all hospitals had more than 15 cases). Figure shows mean score (■) and 95% confidence interval (bar); solid line is mean for all patients; dotted line is median

- Patient completed postal questionnaires are a practical method of obtaining health status information on large samples.
- Generic health status measure can usefully be considered alongside scales specific to conditions.

The effects of this information on changing practice have as yet been limited. The data have prompted questions over practice – for example, the observation that patients with rheumatoid arthritis show as great a benefit as those with osteoarthritis has implications for questions of patient selection. There is concern over why bilateral knee replacements seem worse at three months than unilateral replacements and whether it would be better to spread the two procedures. Addressing these types of questions requires additional analysis of the data.

It is important to consider some reasons why there has been so little practical change. This may be owing to something more general about audit – or the way it was conducted.

It is clear that general health scales have great potential and can be sufficiently sensitive to show change in this client group. They have a great appeal in the breadth of their view of health and in attempting to assess the consequences of care from a patient's perspective.[23] Their disadvantages lie in the problems in interpretation and the link back to clinical practice. The question of attribution, understanding how the process of care affects the observed outcome, seems easier with measures and scales that are traditionally in the clinical domain. It is easier for a clinician to generate ideas about why a poor range of motion is observed than to say why overall mobility is impaired.

The novelty of the outcome measures and the fact that there are no accepted standards for assessment makes it harder to prompt change. There lurks a constant uncertainty over whether an observed poor outcome is the result of suboptimal practice,

---

Data collection in initial Freeman Hospital study and subsequent multihospital audit

Time	Initial data set	Multihospital audit
Before operation	Basic patient details:	
	Age, sex, identifier, etc.	Yes
	Indications for	
	surgery	Yes
	Proposed surgery	Yes
	Previous surgery	Yes
	Nature arthritis	Yes
	Comorbid conditions	Yes
	Initial x ray	No
	Knee score	Yes
	Nottingham Health	
	Profile (patient)	Yes
On discharge	Postoperative complications	Yes (at follow up)
Follow up	Knee score	Yes
(3 months and	Joint loosening	No
1 year)		
	Nottingham Health	
	Profile (patient)	Yes

variability in measurement, or confounding variables. For example, the multihospital audit in figure 7.3 shows clear and statistically significant differences between units X and Q, which prompt questions such as, how much of that difference is due to case type? What aspects of treatment have resulted in apparently better outcomes in hospital Q?

It may be that the approach to quality improvement through audit requires observing the consequences of change in practice to reinforce the audit (and learning) process. The timescales for audit of outcome are longer, making the connection between means and ends that much harder to establish.

Though there is often an interest – indeed, enthusiasm for – outcome measurement, there are uncertainties over how and when outcomes should be used.[24] Do we need to monitor outcome when there are easier and more informative ways to monitor the process of care? The incidence of deep vein thrombosis is a good example of that dilemma; should we monitor deep vein thromboses or the way prophylaxis is used?

Some authors advocate large scale comparative approaches,[25] such as the multihospital audit of knee replacements, which can potentially prompt questions about variability in practice. On the other hand we may be better advised to have less comparability between sites but a closer focus on specific audit or managerial issues. Without trying different approaches to outcome assessment we will not be able to assess the best ways forward.

1 Bardsley M, Coles J. Practical experiences in auditing patient outcomes. *Quality in Health Care* 1992; 1: 124–30.
2 Cleary R. Establishing inter-hospital comparisons of outcomes. *Journal of Quality Assurance in Health Care*. (in press).
3 Nelissen RG, Brand R, Rozing PM. Survivorship analysis in total condylar knee arthroplasty. *J Bone Joint Surg* 1992; 74(A): 383–9.
4 Freund DA, Dittus RS, Fitzgerald J, Heck D. Assessing and improving outcomes: total knee replacement. *Health Services Research* 1990; 25: 723–6.
5 Deyo RA, Unui TS. Towards clinical applications of health status measures. Sensitivity of scales to clinically important changes. *Health Services Research* 1984; 19: 275–89.
6 Insall JN, Hood RW, Flawn LB, Sullivan DJ. A comparison of four models of total knee replacement. *J Bone Joint Surg* 1976; 58A: 754–65.
7 Insall JN, Dorr LD, Scott RD, Scott WN. Rationale of the Knee Society clinical rating system. *Clin Orthopaed* 1989; 248: 13–4.
8 Goldberg VM, Figgie MP, Figgie HE, Heiple KG, Sobel M. Use of a total condylar knee prosthesis for treatment of osteoarthritis and rheumatoid arthritis. *J Bone Joint Surg* 1988; 70A: 802–11.
9 Mohr DN, Silverstein MD, Ilstrup DM, Heit JA, Morrey BF. Venous thromboembolism associated with hip and knee arthroplasty: current prophylactic practice and outcomes. *Mayo Clinic Proc* 1992; 67: 861–70.
10 Wilkin D, Hallam L, Dogget M. *Measures of need and outcome for primary health care.* Oxford: Oxford Medical Publications, 1992.

11 Bowling A. *Measuring health: a review of quality of life measurement scales.* Milton Keynes: Open University Press, 1991.
12 Kantz EM, Harris WJ, Levitsky K, Ware JE, Davis AR. Methods for assessing condition specific and generic functional status outcomes after total knee replacement. *Medical Care* 1992; **30**: MS240-52.
13 Fries J. Towards an understanding of patient outcome measurement. *Arthritis Rheum* 1983; **26**: 697-704.
14 Meenan RF, Gertman PM, Mason JH. Measuring health status in arthritis: the Arthritis Impact Measurement Scales. *Arthritis Rheum* 1980; **23**: 146-52.
15 Bergner M, Bobbitt RA, Carter WB. The Sickness Impact Profile: development and final testing of a health status measure. *Medical Care* 1981; **19**: 787-805.
16 Hunt SM, McEwen J, McKenna SP. *Measuring health status.* Beckenham: Croon Helm, 1986.
17 Jenkinson C, Coulter A, Wright L. Short Form 36 (SF-36) health survey questionnaire: normative data for adults of working age. *BMJ* 1993; **306**: 1437-40.
18 Garratt AM, Ruta DA, Abdalla MI, Buckingham, KJ, Russell IT. The SF 36 health survey questionnaire: an outcome measure suitable for routine use within the NHS? *BMJ* 1993; **306**: 1440-4.
19 Kind P, Carr-Hill R. The Nottingham Health Profile: a useful tool for epidemiologists? *Soc Sci Med* 1987; **25**: 905-10.
20 Jenkinson C, Fitzpatrick R, Argyle M. The Nottingham Health Profile: an analysis of its sensitivity in differentiating illness group. *Soc Sci Med* 1988; **27**: 1411-4.
21 Fitzpatrick R. Surveys of patient satisfaction. I. Important general considerations. *BMJ* 1991; **302**: 887-9.
22 Burton KE, Wright V, Richards J. Patients' expectations in relation to outcome of total hip replacement. *Ann Rheum Dis* 1979; **38**: 471-4.
23 Deyo RA, Patrick DL. Barriers to the use of health status measures in clinical investigation, patient care and policy research. *Medical Care* 1989; **27**(suppl): S254-S268.
24 Epstein AM. The outcomes movement – will it get us where we want to go? *N Engl J Med* 1990; **323**: 266-9.
25 Ellwood PM. Shattuck lecture – outcomes management. A technology of patient experience. *N Engl J Med* 1988; **318**: 1549-56.

8 Routine evaluation of minimally invasive surgery

KLIM McPHERSON

In terms of the general evaluation of minimally invasive surgery a major problem is illustrated by recent research on transurethral resection of the prostate for benign hyperplasia of the prostate. Comparing the operation with watchful waiting suggests that for some patients the choice is finely balanced.[1] Prostatectomy, just like hysterectomy, tonsillectomy, and carotid endarterectomy, shows striking variations in its population based rate, both between neighbouring small areas and between countries.[2] The table, for example, suggests the possibility that the use of a policy of watchful waiting is more common in those areas with low prostatectomy rates.

Table 8.1 International difference in prostatectomy rate (per 100 000 men per year) in the 1980s[3]

Country	Rate
Australia	183
Canada	229
Denmark	234
Ireland	124
The Netherlands	116
New Zealand	191
Norway	238
Sweden	48
United Kingdom	144
United States	308

Evaluating the safety of different methods of treatment

Discussion with urologists and a systematic review of the literature has revealed important and unsettled uncertainties concerning the indications for prostatectomy. Clinicians are faced with two options among men with symptoms of benign hyperplasia of the prostate: to operate during the "early course" of development and so both prevent any deterioration of the condition, and operate when the patient is relatively young; or to delay the operation and reduce the risk and inconvenience of surgery, but also accept a possible deterioration of symptoms and hence the prospect of non-elective surgery at a later time.

Using evidence from the literature and from longitudinal studies it was possible to assess the life expectancy associated with prostatectomy versus watchful waiting. For men with uncomplicated benign hyperplasia of the prostate, average life expectancy is somewhat lower when prostatectomy is chosen instead of watchful waiting.[4] When adjustment was made for quality of life, however, the operation increased the average expectation of quality adjusted life months. Hence the choice depends on the particular preferences of patients: some may prefer the risks of the operation, including risks of incontinence, impotence, and retrograde ejaculation as well as a small risk of death, in order to gain a likely relief of symptoms: others may not wish to take these risks and prefer to put up with the symptoms, at least for the time being.

In parallel with this work, other choices regarding prostatectomy have been investigated: variations in time and place have existed in the conversion from open operations to transurethral surgery. Different urologists introduced transurethral surgery at different times, some in the early 1970s and others not until much later.

In the United States, readmission and death rates can be calculated from Medicare data linked to social security number for most men undergoing prostatectomy. Thus postdischarge outcomes for the two procedures can be compared a long time after the operation.[5] Such unselected information on the long term sequelae of surgery are rare for obvious reasons. These data indicated a higher long term mortality among men receiving the transurethral rather than the open operation.[6] Such a hypothesis generated from observational data can, in principle, be validated only by using randomised studies. However, consolidated practice patterns and (incomplete) contemporary knowledge make such randomised comparison seem unethical.[7, 8]

To proceed scientifically, longitudinal and independent databases in Oxford, Denmark, and Manitoba were analysed to investigate the same hypotheses and in each the same excess mortality was found for transurethral resection of the prostate – a 50% excess mortality in the eight years after surgery.[6] It might be thought that the decision to use a transurethral resection could be made more safely for small prostate glands and perhaps also for patients with more comorbidity. Such selection could lead to an observed higher subsequent mortality for men undergoing transurethral resection independent of the effect of the particular operation. However, the operation itself could also be harmful, compared to open surgery.[9]

Examination of the Manitoba claims data with adjustment for important information on previous medical history and anaesthesiologists' risk categories made no difference to the apparent mortality excess. Moreover, comparing men with benign hyperplasia only and similar men admitted for transurethral and open surgery compared to men admitted for other discretionary surgery continued to confirm the excess. Further work analysing case records in Manitoba in great detail and making more fine statistical adjustments failed to eliminate the excess.[10] Indeed, work in Denmark with detailed case mix adjustment also fails to eliminate the excess.[11] On the other hand, work in Yale has eliminated the apparent effect by adjustment for case mix.[12]

As a consequence of this work the American Urological Association publicly decided to mount a randomised study of treatment for benign hyperplasia of the prostate in which men with large glands will be randomly allocated between transurethral and open surgery. This has yet to happen because the finance and details have not been agreed, but the need is now well understood. In contrast, an editorial in the BMJ stated "The fact that a recent review [by Roos et al[6]] has suggested that transurethral resection of the prostate may not be as good as urologists have claimed does not detract from the important advantages of this technique in treating benign prostatic hyperplasia."[13] Clearly, since it is unethical for clinicians to randomise when they are not uncertain, whether for "legitimate" reasons or not, no randomised study will happen in the United Kingdom soon. However, assessment of new operations like transcervical endometrial ablation, which uses similar technology, will, possibly as a consequence of this experience, be difficult to introduce without rigorous experimental evaluation.[14]

Further cross sectional follow up studies of patients undergoing prostatectomy in the United States, United Kingdom, and Denmark provide insights into the level of symptoms present preoperatively and the changes attributable to the operation.[5, 15] It is fascinating to observe that the average prostate size is larger in the United Kingdom and the prevalence of serious symptoms is higher preoperatively than in the United States. The average level of symptoms and complication postoperatively is, however, much the same in the two countries (unpublished data). The standardised rate of prostatectomy is around twice as high in America, where presumably the indications for surgery are more liberal.

Conclusions

It seems to me that this unsatisfactory state of affairs is in part a consequence of enthusiastic practitioners finding it difficult to step back and worry about the real consequences of their practice style and then to ask whether the resources could be better spent elsewhere.[16] Such questions are always difficult for providers to ask, of course, but in the end they do have to be addressed. The problem with surgery, particularly highly technical interventions like transurethral resection of the prostate, is that the experts (and therefore often the adjudicators of research priorities) are also the enthusiastic providers. However, the Royal College of Surgeons has, since the publication of this work, organised an audit of outcome of 4000 consecutive cases. Observational methods in these circumstances of implied uncertainties only may be more useful than nothing.[17]

1 Wennberg J, Mulley A, Henley D, et al. An assessment of prostatectomy for benign urinary tract obstruction. geographic variations and the evaluation of medical care outcomes. *JAMA* 1988; 259: 3027–30.
2 McPherson K, Wennberg J, Hovind O, Clifford P. Small area variations in the use of common surgical procedures: an international comparison of New England, England and Norway. *N Engl J Med* 1982; 307: 1310–4.

3 McPherson K. International differences in medical care practices. *Health Care Financing Review.* 1989; (Suppl).

4 Barry MJ, Mulley AG, Fowler FJ, Wennberg JE. Watchful waiting versus immediate transurethral resection for symptomatic prostatism: the importance of patients preferences. *JAMA* 1988; **259**: 3010-7.

5 Fowler FJ, Wennberg JE, Timothy RP, Barry MJ, Mulley AG, Henley D, *et al.* Symptom status and the quality of life following prostatectomy. *JAMA* 1988; **259**: 3018-22.

6 Roos NP, Wennberg JE, Malenka DJ, Fisher ES, McPherson K, Anderson TF, *et al.* Mortality and reoperation after open and transurethral resection of the prostate for benign prostatic hyperplasia. *N Engl J Med* 1989; **320**: 1120-4.

7 TU or not TU? *Lancet* 1989; **i**: 1361-2.

8 Baum M. Treatment of benign prostatic hyperplasia *BMJ* 1989; **299**: 979-80.

9 Evans JW, Singer M, Chapple CR, Macartney N, Walker JM, Milroy EJ. Haemodynamic evidence for cardiac stress during transurethral prostatectomy. *BMJ* 1992; **304**: 666-71.

10 Malenka DJ, Roos N, Fisher E, *et al.* Further study of the increased mortality following transurethral prostatectomy: a chart based analysis. *J Urol* 1990; **144**: 224-30.

11 Andersen TF, Bronnum-Hansen H, Sejr T, Roepstorf C. Elevated mortality following transurethral resection of the prostate for benign hypetrrophy! But why? *Medical Care* 1990; **28**: 870-81.

12 Concato J, Horwitz RI, Feinstein AR, Elmore JG, Schiff SF. Problems of comorbidity in mortality after prostatectomy. *JAMA* 1992; **267**: 1077-82.

13 Chisholm GD. Benign prostatic hyperplasia: the best treatment. *BMJ* 1989; **299**: 215-6.

14 Magos AL, Baumann R, Turnbull AC. Transcervical resection of the endometrium in women with menorrhagia *BMJ* 1989; **293**: 1209-12.

15 Flood A, Black N, McPherson K, *et al.* Assessing symptom improvement after elective prostatectomy for benign hypertrophy of the prostate. *Arch Intern Med* 1992; **152**: 1507-12.

16 Chalmers T. Relation of therapeutic advocacy to practice specialty. *JAMA* 1990; **253**: 1392-3.

17 McPherson K. The best and the enemy of the good: randomised controlled trials, uncertainty, and assessing the role of patient choice in medical decision making. The Cochrane Lecture. *J Epidemiol Community Health* 1994; **48**: 6-15.

9 Limitations on the use of cost effectiveness information: ways forward

JAMES RAFTERY

This article argues that cost effectiveness criteria should be applied to the production of information on the cost effectiveness of different health care treatments – more specifically, that the amount and quality of information on cost effectiveness must be informed by its likely cost and benefits, which in turn depend on how that information might be used. David Eddy has suggested four types of limitations to the use of cost effectiveness information – methodological, philosophical, ethical, and clinical.[1-5] The argument presented here extends Eddy's concerns regarding the methodological aspects of cost effectiveness information, using as support, in the context of the reformed NHS, the results of 20 assessments of health needs.

The article suggests three broad ways forward: Firstly, that comparisons within, rather than between, disease offer greater scope for agreeing changes. Lack of precision in estimates of both effectiveness and costs inevitably leaves considerable room for clinical autonomy in decision making at the patient level, with the implication that health gain will be achieved only with the support of clinicians, supported by, rather than led by, contracting. Secondly, the case is made for standardised measures of both effectiveness (health benefit groups) and costs (health care resource groups). Underlying such proposals is the potential for greatly improved information collection and use in health care. Thirdly, the article suggests that the NHS research and development initiative could help by widening its definitions of what constitutes research and by putting more emphasis on development.

Limitations of cost effectiveness information

Recent articles have pointed to the limitations of cost effectiveness league tables on the basis of the poor quality of many studies and of the methodological difficulties involved (discounting, valuation on benefits).[6,7] Other reviews have pointed to the relatively small number of such studies. However, more fundamental limitations apply to cost effectiveness estimates than those outlined in these articles. Estimates of cost effectiveness suffer limitations which become clearer when effectiveness costs are discussed separately.

EFFECTIVENESS

Estimates of effectiveness based on randomised controlled trials are imprecise because of:

(i) being based on samples;
(ii) employing disparate methodologies;
(iii) having a narrow focus;
(iv) being skewed in coverage towards the new;
(v) being constrained in considering older treatments.

There is also

(vi) uncertainty about whose values are counted as benefits, and
(vii) how benefits should be valued over time.

Samples

Randomised controlled trials are based on (often small) sample surveys, picking up only differences in average effectiveness across two groups of people. Interval rather than point estimates result; which, although satisfactory for establishing which treatment works better, are of limited value in quantifying how much better or for which types of patients. Controlling for differences in patient characteristics by randomisation "controls out" much of the information required to establish what Frankel has called "the epidemiology of indications" – that is, who would benefit most from treatment.[8]

Methodologies

Many studies of effectiveness have been characterised by poor methodologies, as indicated by the popularity of meta-analysis and by critiques of the statistical analyses. Meta-analysis shows many studies to have had insufficient power to detect differences, so that only when they are aggregated can differences be detected. The biggest barrier to meta-analysis has to do with disparate methodologies which tend to be incompletely reported. The poor quality of many published medical studies of effectiveness has been the subject of several recent articles.[9, 10]

Narrow focus

The dominance of disease (or often subdisease specific) outcome measurement in effectiveness studies means that, although effectiveness measures can be used to guide policy for the range of treatments within a disease, in the absence of inter-disease measures they can seldom be used across diseases. Yet it is precisely the latter that is required for the use of cost effectiveness information to allocate resources between different diseases.

Skew to the new

Effectiveness studies tend to be skewed to evaluating relatively new treatments. For example, new drugs have had to be evaluated for efficacy and safety in many industrialised countries in the past 20 years. Non-drug therapies are often evaluated by enthusiasts as part of the diffusion of the technology. Popular non-drug therapies tend not to be evaluated, as instanced by the rise of minimally invasive surgery.[11, 12] Further, evaluation tends to be continually out of date because of changing technology.

Limits on the old

Ethical considerations limit the extension of randomised controlled trials to the bulk of older treatment. For example, in the comparison of the effectiveness of limb salvage versus amputation, death could be blamed on the randomisation process preventing what in retrospect might have been the most appropriate treatment.

While these criticisms apply mainly to randomised controlled trials, they also apply in varying degrees to observational studies. Though randomised controlled trials provide good methods of testing interventions, they are costly and time consuming. Observational studies of effectiveness, such as those used in several American patient outcome research teams (PORTs) may offer ways forward, with their costs depending on the extent and validity of clinical information systems. However, doubts have recently been cast on the value of observational studies.[13]

Whose benefits?

Although the health benefit of treatment is conventionally assumed to be that of the patient, in some instances it seems reasonable to include benefits to others, such as carers. As long as benefit is defined purely in health terms, confining its measurement to the patient seems reasonable, but once wider definitions of benefit are considered, such as reassurance, then it becomes more difficult to exclude the benefits to carers.[14]

Benefits over time

The issue of how benefits should be valued over time (the discounting issue) is much more than a technical question in that the relative ranking of the total benefit of some interventions with long time scales, such as those affecting the unborn or the very young, can be altered by the rate at which benefits are discounted over time. The recent controversy in health economics has shown profound disagreement on the topic.[15, 16]

COSTS

Data on costs in most studies are weak for the following reasons:

   (i) definition of costs;
   (ii) costing methods;
   (iii) variations in unit costs, which could be due to many factors (differences in efficiency, case mix, or intensity of treatment).

Cost definitions

The defining of costs in economics as social opportunity costs has both advantages and limitations. The laudable aim of including all the cost effects of a particular intervention (which is observed more in the breach than in the observance), each valued in terms of the next best opportunity foregone, provides endless scope for differences in methodologies and thus contributes largely to the "halfway technology" that has been used to characterise cost effective evaluation.[17] Each study tends to start again rather than be built on shared approaches which might be applied routinely and at low cost. While the direct costs of a unit providing health services can often be obtained from routine sources, data on the indirect costs (such as family care) tend to be expensive as they require sensitive interviews. Recent suggestions that a "restricted list" based on the main cost drivers performs almost as well as more detailed analysis offers promise, but it may apply only to certain diseases.[18]

Secondly, the conventional definition excludes transfer payments (social security payments) despite the possibility that changes in these benefits may be central to the changes of policy being studied. The wisdom here is that transfer payments simply redistribute purchasing power from one group to another, leaving total expenditure unchanged. Housing benefit presents a tricky problem in that the possibility of community based care can depend on the rules governing housing benefit. For example, social security payments for many resettled mental health patients go directly to the agency providing the accommodation rather than to the patient (who might spend it on other things). Since the housing benefit may never reach the hands of the recipient, it should perhaps be treated as a cost that would not otherwise have been incurred. Cost comparisons of community versus hospital care that ignore hotel costs in the former but count them in the latter are not comparing like with like.

Costing methods

The total costs of a service depend on the number of units of service provided and the unit costs of each of these. Neither tend to be well defined in the NHS. The units in which services are measured varies widely, from episodes of care to inpatient days in the acute inpatient sector, with contacts (first and total) used in the primary care and community services. None of these proxies can be relied on to pick up "true" costs, certainly not without validation. Progress in defining health care products that cost on average the same has been slow, but diagnosis related groups in the United States and more recently health care resource groups (HRGs) in the United Kingdom[19] define standard inpatient products by combining cases based on diagnosis and procedure with patient characteristics such as age and comorbidities so that each case falling into one of these groups can be expected to cost roughly the same. Extension of this approach to ambulatory and long term care would seem to be the next stage, following the American experience. For these groups to work, however, outliers (those with values very different from the average in the group) have to be excluded. Studies which do not use a standard product definition in costing services run the risk of attributing difference to averages rather than to exceptional outliers. Very few studies have used standard products in their costing, and the degree to which cost differences are due to outliers remains unknown.

Even where the right product is costed, a variety of cost definitions can be used, depending on the time scale, with short run marginal cost changes likely to differ from long run marginal costs (the latter approximating to average cost). Although economic theory favours use of both short run and long run marginal costs, these are seldom available in practice. Many studies use average costs, thus implicitly overstating the cost changes that will occur in the short run.

Variations in unit costs

Wide variations exist in unit costs, whether measured at the level of cost per finished consultant episode or inpatient day, by specialty, or by subspecialty group. These variations are difficult to interpret because they could be due to many factors, such as differences in technical efficiency, in case mix, in intensity of treatments, or in costing methods (such as treatment of outliers). Most estimates of costs assume full technical efficiency – that is, that inputs are being combined in ways which generate the maximum output, a somewhat heroic assumption in a context that has traditionally lacked incentives to be technically efficient. These assumptions have the premise that the hospital behaves as a commercial firm might. While the problems of making such assumptions are known,[20] nothing is known about how hospitals function as organisations. Many British hospitals have resembled loose confederations rather than unified entities, with many small clinical firms acting in isolation. The move to NHS trusts may shift hospitals towards behaving more like commercial firms, but the degrees of freedom and risk they are allowed to undertake remain matters of some contention.

PRODUCTIVE EFFICIENCY

The issue of efficiency in health care provision raises a further set of questions. The distinction between allocative and productive efficiency is important. Allocative efficiency refers to the optimal allocation of resources between sectors, here referring to health care interventions or services. Cost effectiveness estimates are often aimed at improving allocative efficiency (such as providing more hip replacements at the cost of fewer heart transplants). Productive or technical efficiency refers to the degree that inputs are combined to maximise outputs (or, given output, inputs are minimised). Although productive efficiency is conventionally assumed in market based organisations (based on the notion that people tend to maximise in their self interest), it cannot always be assumed, particularly if organisational structures limit what they can maximise.[21] More specifically, it cannot readily be assumed in a health care system such as the NHS which has traditionally lacked incentives for such behaviour. The fact that money did not follow the patient was one of the mainsprings of the NHS reforms. Pay levels were not linked to performance, and so on. Changing technology means that the efficiency boundary is continually shifting so that achievement of productive efficiency would require continual changes in work practices. Yet most studies assume that the bit of the NHS they are studying is productively efficient.

The implications of possibly different levels of productive efficiency are considerable in that comparisons of apparent cost differences may not be comparing like with like. The necessity for local exploration of costs is underlined, and may well be an onus on the purchaser as well as on the providers. Finally, it is arguable that efforts to achieve greater productive efficiency within diseases should take precedence over issues of allocative efficiency between diseases.

COST EFFECTIVENESS

The weaknesses in both the information on effectiveness and on costs combine to limit cost effectiveness estimates in the following ways:

(i) imprecise estimates;

(ii) micro focus.

Imprecise estimates

Cost effectiveness estimates, by combining effectiveness and costs in a single quotient, amplify the imprecision in each for several reasons. Firstly, in purely statistical terms, the error terms are additive, which causes the confidence intervals to expand. Consider an effectiveness estimate with confidence interval of ±10% and a similar range for the cost estimate. The confidence interval of the combined estimates is approximately ±20%. Secondly, while the effectiveness of a treatment may be similar in different places for well defined patients, in practice the types of patients treated, the amount of service used per patient, and the unit costs involved may well differ by place. Thus cost effectiveness estimates based on one location may be specific to that location and applicable to other locations only with suitable adjustments. Sensitivity analysis is required on both numerator and denominator of the cost effectiveness estimate and should also explore the components of total cost - namely, the quantity of service and the unit price - as well as the treatment of outliers.

Confidence intervals around cost effectiveness estimates are rare, however, partly for the reasons discussed above, which lead to cost estimates often being poorly reported. Similar problems apply to power calculations, which in most studies are based on the likely differences in effectiveness rather than on costs. Ideally, differences in both effectiveness and cost should be taken into account in studies designed to establish cost effectiveness.

The result is that cost effectiveness estimates should only be taken as indicating orders of magnitude. Rather than QALY league tables, division of such estimates into leagues may be more appropriate, since what matters is what division a treatment falls into. For example, the use of six divisions such as cost per QALY of <£1000, through four intermediate divisions to >£50 000 makes more intuitive sense than do the continuous variables that are usually reported, which imply a spurious accuracy.

Micro focus

The methodological problems to do with cost effectiveness estimates mean that greater caution should be exercised in making comparisons between different studies and between different diseases than within a single study. While micro or within disease comparisons of effectiveness can often be made, the lack of a generic measure of effectiveness and the possibility of different methodologies inhibit comparisons between diseases. Within disease comparisons that trade off morbidity and mortality raise the ethical issues familiar to observers of the QALY debate. This point is picked up in the third part of this article, which suggests a restricted focus on within disease comparisons.

Both micro and macro measures of cost effectiveness suffer methodological deficiencies to do with quality of life valuations and their treatment over time. Technically, to be helpful in making decisions about marginal changes, marginal estimates of cost effectiveness are required, based on appropriately scaled measures. The main contenders for such a generic measure of cost effectiveness, such as quality adjusted life years (QALYs), disability adjusted life years (DALYs),[22] and well years,[23] all suffer limitations to do with the number of dimensions, the weighting of different states, discounting of benefits and the timescale for the measure of life years.

Overall, it can be concluded that the lack of methodological agreement on many issues to do with the measurement of both outcomes and costs will prevent the graduation of cost effectiveness evaluation from its "halfway technology" status for some time. The next section considers the degree to which this finding was borne out by a health needs assessment programme which reviewed 20 diseases.

Cost effectiveness information and the epidemiological health needs assessment programme

The result of an epidemiological health needs assessment programme that commissioned reviews against a common protocol provides a summary review of what is known about effectiveness and cost effectiveness of treatments in 20 diseases/topics.[24] The focus on diseases and their treatments from a population perspective characterised the programme, which was sponsored by the NHS Executive. The protocol included the prevalence and incidence of the disease, the services available, and the effectiveness and cost effectiveness of those services.

In a concluding review of the 20 studies, the editors considered the degree to which the mixture of services available broadly matched what was known about their relative effectiveness.[25] They suggested that three types could be distinguished:

(i) Diseases whose pattern of services was broadly supported by evidence (9 topics: renal disease, 6 elective surgical topics, lower respiratory disease, family planning/abortion/infertility);

(ii) Diseases whose mix of services had mixed evidence (8 topics: colorectal cancer, adult mental health services, coronary heart disease, people with learning disabilities, dementia, alcohol abuse, drug abuse); and

(iii) Diseases whose mix of services had a core mismatch with the evidence (3 topics: lung cancer, stroke, community child health services).

The reports on the diseases falling into category (i) tended to explore the implication of meeting need (defined as ability to benefit), while those in (ii) and (iii) variously advocated improved coordination (3 diseases), a shift to prevention (3), or other changes.

Each study highlighted serious information deficiencies not only in relation to cost effectiveness but also to do with levels of service use and cost. Where procedures were known to be effective, such as in elective surgery, little or nothing was known about the extent to which the most appropriate patients were being treated. Hence the concern with an epidemiology of indications – indications, that is, of which types of patients would benefit most. Questions of this sort raise the fundamental methodological complexities discussed above.

Overall, the health needs assessment revealed the degree to which health services are provider led rather than purchaser led. For some diseases, the mix of services provided seems simply to be wrong. For others, when the right services are provided, we do not know if the right amounts are being provided to the right people. The ideal of basing purchasing decisions on comprehensive information on the relative cost effectiveness of every treatment by patient type makes the economics of health an unusually dismal science! Yet despite the information deficiencies, each of the health needs assessments was able to make a plausible case for the direction if not the magnitude of the changes required.

Ways forward

There are three broad ways forward:

- A focus for cost effectiveness comparisons within diseases or client groups is more appropriate than cross disease comparisons;
- Scope exists for developing standardised measures of effectiveness as well as those on costs (health care resource groups), and these could be linked to give rough overall measures of cost effectiveness;
- These directions have implications for research and development.

A NARROWER FOCUS ON DISEASES OR CLIENT GROUPS

A focus on diseases or client groups has a number of advantages. Firstly, it offers ways of combining local information on costs and productive efficiency with epidemiological knowledge of effectiveness as well as on the prevalence and incidence of diseases and conditions. Secondly, the lack of precision in estimates of effectiveness and costs leaves considerable room for involving clinicians both in the quest for productive efficiency and in acknowledging the inevitability of clinical autonomy in decisionmaking at the patient level. Greater understanding of the potential role and limitations of the use of cost effectiveness information would also mark a step forward both in discouraging inappropriate use of cost effectiveness information and in identifying the most useful research.

Acknowledgment that purchasing health care is never going to be like shopping in the supermarket is important, if only because some seem to see it in such terms.[26] The nature of the health care product, with its associated information asymmetries and highly personalised nature, means that clinicians will always be the key decision makers. Purchasers will not be able to influence clinical practice without winning the minds of (most) clinicians. Making clinicians aware of the cost and effectiveness implications of their

95

decisions offers an immediate way forward, which may or may not lead to changes. Improved monitoring of clinical behaviour linked to audit can clearly help. To the degree that health authorities as purchasers occupy the "high moral ground" in terms of health gain, they may be able to escape the damaging perception of their role as cost cutters.

A narrower focus on diseases or client groups seems to offer a way of combining local information on costs and productive efficiency with epidemiological knowledge of effectiveness as well as on the prevalence and incidence of diseases and conditions. Local information is essential if issues to do with costs and the productive efficiency of suppliers are to be addressed. Knowledge of effectiveness is valuable partly because it has a much wider coverage than that on cost effectiveness. For example, a search of Medline 1981–93 under "effectiveness" yields 20 000 references, while one on "cost effectiveness" yields only one tenth of that number. More importantly, effectiveness information is likely to be more generalisable than cost effectiveness information, because of variations in costs by locality. Knowledge of prevalence and incidence can be useful in assessing the magnitudes of potential demand; if broken down by appropriate subcategories it can indicate the likely level of need (defined as ability to benefit). Rather than an epidemiology of aetiology (the conventional approach), what is required is an "epidemiology of indications"[8] which distinguishes between patients in terms of ability to benefit.

STANDARDISED MEASURES OF EFFECTIVENESS AND COSTS

The lack of standardised measures of effectiveness and of costs, as well as the large number of estimates required to cover the range of health care interventions, suggests that there is value in developing such standardised measures. This approach, which is explored in chapter 14 in this volume, would give a two dimensional grid with costs on one axis and effectiveness on the other within which to locate treatments. Such a grid could acknowledge the imprecision of both effectiveness and cost estimates and provide scope for use of local costs. The resulting broad estimates of cost effectiveness might be useful for comparative purposes as well as to identify those services requiring further investigation because of seemingly high or low cost effectiveness. They would need order of magnitude estimates in purchasing – a map of the country rather than street maps of parts of it. The large number of treatments – perhaps 15 000 different types of hospital treatment; more if personal characteristics of patients are taken into account – means that some grouping of treatments is essential.

Implications for research and development

The first implication for research and development is that we need more development, less research. Examples include improved use of existing data on variations in practice, more integrated information on effectiveness and patterns of service use. Secondly, an acceptance that effectiveness and costs can be derived separately, rather than every study having to include both, could be useful. Thirdly, studies should include a range of resource measures, including levels of service use and unit costs, to enable local validation, sensitivity analysis, etc. Fourthly, studies should include a range of measures of effectiveness, with exchange rates to enable different levels of aggregation for use in different contexts. Finally, the improved use of cost effectiveness information in the health services should perhaps best be seen as a labour of Sisyphus, which will never be completed. More clarity about likely use and limitations may ease the task.

1 Eddy DM. Clinical decision making: from theory to practice. Applying cost-effectiveness analysis. The inside story. *JAMA* 1992; **268:** 2575–82.
2 Eddy DM. Clinical decision making: from theory to practice. Cost-effectiveness analysis. Will it be accepted? *JAMA* 1992; **268:** 132–6.
3 Eddy DM. Clinical decision making: from theory to practice. Cost-effectiveness analysis. Is it up to the task? *JAMA* 1992; **267:** 3342–8.
4 Eddy DM. Clinical decision making: from theory to practice. Cost-effectiveness analysis. A conversation with my father. *JAMA* 1992; **267:** 1669–75.
5 Eddy DM. Oregon's methods. Did cost-effectiveness analysis fail? *JAMA* 1991; **266:** 2135–41.
6 Mason J, Drummond M, Torrance G. Some guidelines on the use of cost effectiveness league tables. *BMJ* 1993; **306:** 570–2.
7 Drummond M, Torrance G, Mason J. Cost-effectiveness league tables: more harm than good? *Soc Sci Med* 1993; **37:** 33–40.
8 Frankel SJ. The epidemiology of indications. *J Epidemiol Community Health* 1991; **45:** 257–9.
9 Altman D. The scandal of medical research. *BMJ* 1994; **308:** 283–4.
10 Williamson JW, Goldschmidt PF, Colton T. The quality of medical literature: an analysis of validation assessments. In: Bailar JC, Mosteller F, eds. *Medical uses of statistics.* Waltham, MA.: NEJM Books, 1986; 151–75.
11 Banta HD. The cost-effectiveness of 10 selected applications in minimally invasive therapy. *Health Policy* 1993; **23:** 135–51.
12 Banta HD. Introduction. Minimally invasive therapy in five European countries: diffusion, effectiveness and cost-effectiveness. *Health Policy* 1993; **23:** 1–5.
13 Sheldon T. Please bypass the PORT. *BMJ* 1994; **309:** 142–3.

14 Orchard C. Comparing healthcare outcomes. *BMJ* 1994; **308**: 1493–6.
15 Parsonage M, Neuberger H. Discounting and QALYs. *Health Economics* 1992; 1: 71–9.
16 Sheldon AT. Discounting in health care decision-making: time for a change? *J Public Health Med* 1992; **14**: 250–6.
17 Hutton J. Cost-benefit analysis in health care expenditure decision-making. *Health Econ* 1992; 1: 213–6.
18 Knapp M, Beecham J. Reduced list costings: examination of an informed short cut in mental health research. *Health Econ* 1993; 2: 313–22.
19 Sanderson H. Measuring case mix. *BMJ* 1992; **304**: 1067–8.
20 McGuire A. The theory of the hospital: a review of the models. *Soc Sci Med* 1985; **20**: 1177–84.
21 Milgrom P, Roberts J. *Economics, organisation and management.* New Jersey: Prentice-Hall, 1992.
22 *World Bank development report 1993 – investing in health.* Oxford: Oxford University Press, 1994.
23 Kaplan RM, Bush JW, Bury CC. Health related quality of life measurement for evaluation research and policy analysis. *Health Psychology* 1982; 1: 61.
24 Stevens A, Raftery J, eds. *Health care needs assessment – the epidemiologically based need assessment reviews.* Oxford: Radcliffe Medical Press, 1994.
25 Raftery J, Stevens A. Reflections and conclusions. In: Stevens A, Raftery J, eds. *Health care needs assessment – the epidemiologically based needs assessment reviews.* Vol   Oxford: Radcliffe Medical Press, 1994, 595–623.
26 Dawson D. *Costs and prices in the internal market: markets versus the NHS Management Executive guidelines.* York: Centre for Health Economics, 1994; (Discussion Paper 115).

10 How should information on cost effectiveness influence clinical practice?

ALAN WILLIAMS

Information on cost effectiveness should influence clinical practice through practice guidelines, monitored within clinical audit, and reinforced by purchasers through the contractual process. In principle there should be no resistance to this. After all, the objective of cost effectiveness analysis is to ensure that the limited resources at our disposal are used to bring about the maximum improvement in people's health, and that is also the objective of clinical audit and the objective of purchasers.

Moreover, various official bodies involved in this area of activity have stated their positions in an encouraging way.

In a recent booklet entitled The Evolution of Clinical Audit[3] the Department of Health cites one of its earlier publications[4] as providing "the strategic direction for clinical audit": "Clinical audit involves systematically looking at the procedures used for diagnosis, care and treatment, examining how associated resources are used and investigating the effect care has on the outcome and quality of life for the patient."

Unfortunately the booklet then departs significantly from this remit by ignoring resources completely, except for resources devoted to the audit process itself. More recently still, the NHS Management Executive sent round an Executive Letter which includes a section on the use of clinical guidelines to inform the contracting process. It states that such guidelines will need to be

- developed and endorsed by the relevant professional bodies
- based on good research evidence of clinical effectiveness
- practical and affordable
- where appropriate, multidisciplinary, and
- take account of patient choices and values.[5]

It is well known that the road to hell is paved with good intentions, and consensual agreement in principle is no guarantee that things will actually turn out the way that well intentioned people wish. Some of the difficulties are purely practical, and the greatest practical difficulty in this field is lack of relevant information. Superficially, there are plenty of data (that is, facts untouched by human thought) about the conduct of clinical practice, but most of them cannot be applied systematically even to the issues which the creation of narrowly focused clinical guidelines brings to the fore, let alone to the issues which a cost effectiveness approach brings to the fore.

But there is a prior problem which I fear will misdirect attempts to fill the information void if we are not aware of it. The problem in question is that many of those who pay lip service to the need for clinical practice to be pursued in a cost effective way do not really appreciate what they are committing themselves to, and they tend to shrink from the implications when they realise what they are.

I have written elsewhere about the weaknesses of clinical audit (as typically practised in the United Kingdom) as a mechanism for checking that clinicians behave in a cost effective way.[6] Instead of commenting on the currently rather tentative use by purchasers of the latent power that they have to redirect clinical activity into more cost effective channels, I will concentrate on the potential role of practice guidelines in this matter.

It has been suggested that purchasers should not be buying "treatments" but "treatment protocols" (which I am here calling "practice guidelines"). The idea is that when a patient presents, the case is identified as falling within a particular guideline, and a particular protocol is then followed. This may lead to an expensive treatment being offered or to no treatment being offered, depending on what happens as the protocol is followed. The purchaser pays a fixed sum of money for each presenting case; this takes account of all these possibilities and does not depend on the actual treatment offered to any particular patient. It would be monitored for all presenting cases (by random sampling perhaps) through clinical audit to ensure that the protocol was properly followed. It is against that scenario that I wish to consider the problem of ensuring that these guidelines are drawn up appropriately.

My starting point is a recently published book from the Royal College of Physicians of London called Analysing How We Reach Clinical Decisions.[7] The introduction states:

> It is important ... to be able to analyse the reasoning process which leads to diagnoses and decisions on clinical management. The discipline which addresses this issue is called "clinical decision analysis," and draws on a number of other disciplines, especially probability theory and the assessment of "utility" or "value" of outcomes of medical intervention.

A little later an important caveat appears:

> The decision about how to deal with a particular patient may be made from different points of view. It is entirely the patient's point of view which will be considered in this introductory book. In the United Kingdom, most patients do not have to take the cost of care into consideration .... A decision can also be considered from a hospital or departmental manager's point of view. For example, if a limited number of beds is available, a priority decision may have to be made as to who should be admitted. A doctor may have to make a decision which combines both points of view. Decision analysis allows decisions of this kind to be made explicit.

It is on the implications of this last sentence that I wish to elaborate.

An example

Let us take a very simple clinical decision problem (figure 10.1). For a particular class of presenting signs and symptoms, a diagnostic test will generate two results, A or B. If the result is A, two alternative treatments (X and Y) are commonly offered; if the result is B, two alternative treatments (Y and Z) are commonly offered. Each of the three treatments has a "good" and a "bad" outcome, with known probability. The clinical problem is: given the test result, which treatment should be offered?

101

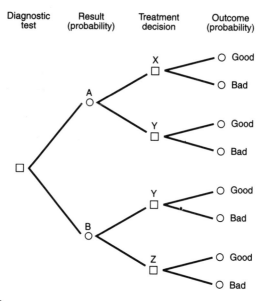

Figure 10.1

Some basic data is supplied in figure 10.2. This comprises the respective probabilities associated with the two test results, and the probabilities associated with each outcome for each treatment. There is also a quantitative indicator of the amount of health gain for each outcome. To keep things simple, this can be thought of as additional years of life, but it might be quality adjusted life years or some other measure of benefit appropriate to the situation. When these health gains for each outcome are multiplied by the probability of getting that outcome we arrive at the "expected" health gain, which when summed for each treatment (that is, across the good and bad outcomes for that treatment) gives us the "expected" benefit from the treatment. For the alternative treatments on offer when the test result is A, treatment Y offers greater expected benefits than treatment X, and should therefore be chosen. Similar reasoning will lead to treatment Z being chosen when the test result is B.

The basic approach

Figure 10.2 is an example of the class of decisions analysed in the basic texts on clinical decision making, and it is this same class of decisions that is analysed in the Royal College of Physicians'

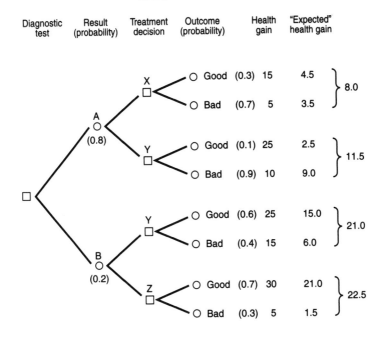

Diagnostic test	Result (probability)	Treatment decision	Outcome (probability)	Health gain	"Expected" health gain

Decisions: If test result is A, offer treatment Y
If test result is B, offer treatment Z

Figure 10.2

book.[7] The weakness of this analysis is that it pays no regard to the costs of treatment, being wholly concerned with "effectiveness." This renders such a guideline or protocol deeply suspect from a purchaser's viewpoint, and is in my view irresponsible even from a clinician's viewpoint. As I have argued elsewhere, clinicians, like purchasers, have responsibilities to a whole group of patients and potential patients, which they can discharge responsibly only by taking into account the consequences for resource use which flow from their decisions (for example the use of the hospital beds or operating theatre time that has been allocated to them).[8] Figure 10.2 ignores that consideration.

There is a temptation at this stage to repair the weaknesses in the "effectiveness only" approach by throwing in some cost data, almost as an afterthought. In more complex situations than that shown in figure 10.2, this would be an enormous task if every alternative branch and twig in a dense decision tree had to be

103

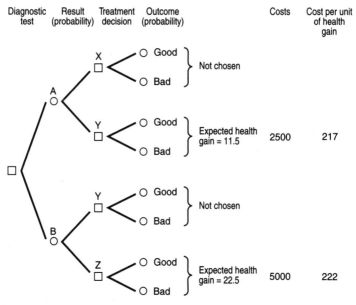

Figure 10.3

properly costed, so what tends to happen is that only the chosen options are costed, just to check that they are "affordable." This implies that the decision problem is seen as the one shown in figure 10.3, where the cost per unit of health gain for the two chosen treatments has been added to the previous analysis. If 217 and 222 are "acceptable" cost levels (if, for example, many other treatments being offered elsewhere in the system exceed this level of cost per unit of health gain) then the clinical seal of approval is fixed to the protocol, and it is henceforth claimed to be the cost effective procedure, and recommended on those grounds.

A turnaround

In the more advanced texts on clinical decision analysis these problems are dealt with by integrating the cost data into the decision tree itself, in the manner shown in figure 10.4.[9, 10] This ignores the costs of the test itself, though in a more broad ranging review they would have to be included. The costs that have been added are the costs associated with each treatment option, and they have been carefully selected to make a point. When the cost per unit of health gain is calculated for all four options, neither of

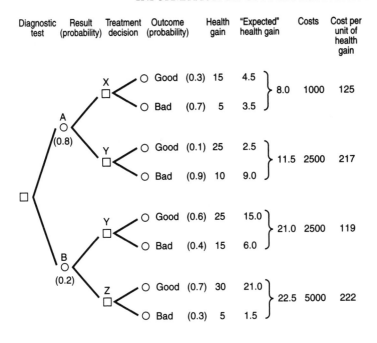

Diagnostic test	Result (probability)	Treatment decision	Outcome (probability)		Health gain	"Expected" health gain	Costs	Cost per unit of health gain
		X	Good	(0.3) 15	4.5	8.0	1000	125
			Bad	(0.7) 5	3.5			
A (0.8)								
		Y	Good	(0.1) 25	2.5	11.5	2500	217
			Bad	(0.9) 10	9.0			
		Y	Good	(0.6) 25	15.0	21.0	2500	119
			Bad	(0.4) 15	6.0			
B (0.2)								
		Z	Good	(0.7) 30	21.0	22.5	5000	222
			Bad	(0.3) 5	1.5			

Decisions: If test result is A, offer treatment X
If test result is B, offer treatment Y

Figure 10.4

the previous recommendations holds. When the test result is A, it is now treatment X that is recommended rather than treatment Y, and when the test result is B it is now Y that is indicated, not Z. So the really cost effective procedure is the opposite to what was mistakenly claimed at the end of the preceding paragraph.

Let us pause to consider the implications of this turnaround. It means that patients with this condition are not being offered the "best" treatment, if by "best" we mean the one that would do each of them the most good. How can this be justified? Let us do some more arithmetic. In the "effectiveness only" scenario in figures 10.2 or 10.3, the average cost per presenting patient is 3000 (see appendix). The corresponding figure in the "cost effectiveness" scenario in figure 10.4 is 1300. With resources available for these patients amounting to £300 000 a year, under the "effectiveness only" scenario 100 patients could be treated each year, whereas under the cost effectiveness scenario 231 could be

105

treated. So although each treated patient gets a greater expected benefit under the "effectiveness only" protocol (13.7 v 10.6), the total benefit is much greater under the cost effectiveness protocol (2449 v 1370) because many more patients get treated.

Conclusions

We are brought back to the question: what objective are we pursuing? Is it "clinical excellence" (no matter what the costs?) or ensuring that the people we serve are as healthy as it is possible for us to make them, given the resources (human and material) available to us?" If we all share the "healthy" objective, then purchasers, clinicians, and decision analysts need to get together

---

Views of cost effectiveness analysis

Royal College of Physicians:

> More systematic evaluation of the quality and effectiveness of doctor's work ... can now be regarded as an important professional obligation....
>
> Adequate audit should measure quality as well as quantity of care. The measurement of quality is ... difficult ... because ... a patient and doctor may well have different views ....
>
> Ideally, review should include both clinical outcome and cost: unnecessarily extravagant practices used for some patients deprive others of their appropriate share.[1]

Royal College of Surgeons of England:

> Audit is the systematic appraisal of the implementation and outcome of any process in the context of prescribed targets and standards. Clinical audit is the process by which medical staff collectively review, evaluate and improve their practice. This should include
> - the access of patients to care ...
> - the process and outcome of care
> - the administrative and financial constraints relevant to clinical practice....
>
> Clinical audit meetings should address a variety of topics
> a) Access to treatment ...
> b) Issues. The appropriateness and complications of clinical investigations of treatment, the use of resources ... should all be addressed
> c) Outcomes.[2]

---

to devise clinical guidelines that embody the cost effectiveness approach to health care. Only in that way will we achieve the ambitions of the august bodies whose views were cited at the outset, and who emphasised the need to be systematic and to take into account both resource use and patient outcome (in terms of survival and of quality of life). But I fear that if this is to happen in my lifetime a rather more fundamental culture shift is going to be required among clinicians at grass roots level in the United Kingdom than is evident at present, despite the pioneering efforts of the enlightened few. It is in the creation, dissemination, monitoring, and purchasing of truly cost effective treatment protocols that the commitment of the medical profession to this enterprise is about to be tested. I hesitate to predict which way it will go.

Appendix: Calculations for results in the text

In figure 10.3, 80% of patients get treatment A, which costs 2500, and 20% get treatment Z, which costs 5000, so the (weighted) average cost is 0.8 of 2500 (ie, 2000) plus 0.2 of 5000 (ie, 1000), which amounts to 3000 in all. The corresponding figures for the scenario presented in figure 10.4 are 80% getting treatment X (costing 1000 each) and 20% getting treatment Y (costing 2500 each). This generates a weighted average cost of 0.8 of 1000 (ie, 800) plus 0.2 of 2500 (ie, 500), which comes to 1300 in all.

A budget of 300 000 will thus enable 100 patients to be treated if the policy is as set out in figure 10.3, but 231 (300 000/1300) can be treated if the policy is as set out in figure 10.4.

The average benefit from treatment under each scenario can be calculated in a similar manner. In figure 10.3 it is 0.8 of 11.5 plus 0.2 of 22.5 (which comes to 13.7 in all), whereas in figure 10.4 it is 0.8 of 8 plus 0.2 of 21 (which comes to 10.6).

Putting together the benefit per patient and the number of patients treated under each scenario, we have, for figure 10.3, 100 times 13.7 (or 1370) and for figure 10.4, 231 times 10.6 (or 2449).

1 Royal College of Physicians of London. *First report on medical audit*. London: RCP, 1989.
2 Royal College of Surgeons of England. *Guidelines to clinical audit in surgical practice*. London: RCSE, 1989.
3 NHS Management Executive. *The evolution of clinical audit*. Leeds: NHSME, [1993].
4 NHS Management Executive. *Clinical audit: meeting and improving standards in health care*. Leeds: NHSME, 1993.
5 NHS Management Executive. *Improving clinical effectiveness*. Leeds: NHSME, 1993. (EL(93)115).
6 Williams A. Quality assurance from the perspective of health economics. *Proceedings of the Royal Society of Edinburgh* 1993; 101B: 105–14.
7 Llewelyn H, Hopkins A. *Analysing how we reach clinical decisions*. London: Royal College of Physicians, 1993.
8 Williams A. Health economics: the end of clinical freedom? *BMJ* 1988; **297**: 1183–6.
9 Weinstein MC, Fineberg HV. *Clinical decision analysis*. Philadelphia: W B Saunders, 1980.
10 Williams A. The role of economics in the evaluation of health care technologies. In: Culyer AJ, Horisberger B, eds. *Economic and medical evaluation of health care technologies*. Berlin: Springer, 1983: 47–80.

11 What can comparisons of hospital death rates tell us about the quality of care?

MARTIN McKEE, DUNCAN HUNTER

In 1993 the *Times* published a table of postoperative death rates from hospitals throughout England that drew attention to substantial variations after general surgical operations.[1] The *Times* quoted an expert as saying that "going into hospital for a general surgical operation is a game of chance in which some patients lose their lives."

Recent interest in comparisons of quality of care, which hospital death rates at first sight may seem to measure, has arisen for several reasons. All industrialised countries have seen a much greater degree of consumerism in recent years and people quite reasonably wish to know much more about the services that they are receiving. In Britain, the reform of the NHS has highlighted the importance of information in making a market work in health care. In any market, high quality information is essential to avoid market failure.

The first health service league tables do not contain measures of clinical performance. However, a working group of the Joint Consultants Committee and NHS Executive is reviewing the future of performance tables and is considering whether to publish league tables of death rates. The experience in other areas of social policy, such as education, is that the coverage is expanded in subsequent revisions, and it is quite possible that hospital death rates will be published. Indeed, calls for this to happen have featured strongly in initial responses to the publication of the tables. If such league tables are to be published, caution must be used in their interpretation. Fundamental epidemiological issues must be considered; these include confounding, bias, sampling, accuracy, scope for manipulation, and interpretation.

Confounding

The first issue, confounding, relates to the question of whether differences between hospitals or physicians are due solely to clinical performance or could be explained by other factors such as differences in the severity of disease in patients treated. If severity is important can it be adjusted for adequately?

There is clear evidence that severity, defined in various ways such as the probability of complications or death or an increased length of stay, varies considerably between hospitals. Several American tools are available that seek to adjust for differences in severity,[2] including Disease Staging, MedisGroups and Patient Management Categories.

In a study that examined data from all acute hospitals in North West Thames region during a two year period, the observed death rate from cholecystitis in different hospitals varied from 0 to 1.52%.[3] After adjustment for a range of factors including the severity of the disease, measured with Disease Staging;[4] coexisting diseases; age; and method of admission, the expected rate varied from 0.1% to 1.33%. The corresponding figures for observed death rates from ischaemic heart disease varied from 2.23% to 17.76% but the expected rates varied from 0.93% to 6.68%. Clearly a crude comparison of death rates would be completely misleading.

Although systems based on routine data can adjust, to some extent, for differences in severity, there is evidence that they cannot do so completely. Studies comparing, firstly, coronary artery bypass grafting and angioplasty[5, 6] and, secondly, open and transurethral prostatectomy[7–10] show that even quite sophisticated forms of severity adjustment can give misleading results, suggesting that there are real differences when none actually exist. Much better adjustment for severity can be achieved with some systems that use much more detailed information. An example is APACHE II, developed for predicting outcome in intensive care units, which has high power to predict mortality and act as a basis for comparing clinical performance.[11] There is, however, a trade off between detail and cost.

Bias

Bias may arise if the data on which comparisons are based are inaccurate and thus do not represent the true situation. The topic of data accuracy has been examined at length elsewhere. There is clearly a problem, but it may have been overstated because of publication bias.[12]

There is a more fundamental issue concerned with our understanding of the concept of data accuracy. Most studies examine the extent to which observed codes agree with those assigned by experts who look at the notes subsequently. There is an implicit assumption that experts can provide the gold standard. This ignores the limitations of the ICD-9 classification system.[13] It is often difficult to define when a disease is present. To take a common example, the term benign prostatic hypertrophy is commonly used, but urologists cannot agree as to whether it relates to the size of the prostate gland, the extent to which the prostate gland causes urinary symptoms, or extent to which it interferes with urinary flow.[14] This problem faces all coding systems and is not solved by some of the newer approaches such as Read codes.

Bias arises from systematic differences in the way that data are recorded. There are three key questions: are episodes the same as people? does it matter if the data are incomplete? and are differences in lengths of stay important when assessing outcome?

Although there is often a close correlation between episodes and individual patients, the figures may vary considerably with, in some cases, a death rate based on episodes up to 50% less than that based on patients.[3] It is not, however, clear that using people as a denominator is always the correct approach, especially in the case of, for example, someone with more than one disease.

Bias can arise if data are incomplete and those data that are available differ from those that are not. Historically, many hospitals failed to record up to 40% of cases. Although this has improved greatly since information has been required for contracting, up to 10% of cases are still unrecorded in some hospitals. There is evidence from several studies, especially those looking at data from cancer registries, that case notes of patients who die are systematically less likely to be coded and recorded on patient administration systems.[15, 16] This will produce an artificially low apparent death rate.

Bias may also arise from differences in lengths of stay. At present, rates of in hospital mortality are measured rather than those based on either fixed or disease specific time periods. The limitations of this measure are seen from a comparison that shows that the in hospital mortality in California is substantially lower than in New York but the length of stay in California is also much shorter. Following people up after they leave hospital shows that the 30 day mortality is identical. The apparently lower in hospital mortality in California is thus entirely due to the tendency to discharge people home to die rather than keeping them in hospital.[17]

Sample size

The third issue is the effect of sample size. In comparisons of clinical performance, are the numbers of deaths or other adverse outcomes involved sufficiently large to be meaningful or can differences be explained by chance? There are several ways of tackling the effects of small numbers. One is to treat death rates in a particular period as samples in time and calculate confidence intervals.[18] The second, described by Palmer, is to look at the rankings of hospitals during different time periods and calculate a measure of the degree of surprise if one hospital appears in the top or bottom ranking consistently.[19]

Even in data collected over a period of several years and for common conditions, the confidence intervals are often very wide[3] and it is rarely possible to exclude the effect of chance.[20] Although long time periods are often necessary to obtain figures that approach some degree of statistical significance, it is questionable how useful it is to look at data that are, by the time they are analysed, three or more years out of date.

Scope for manipulation

Perhaps the most important issue in the present context is the scope for manipulation. If data are to be published and used as a basis for decisions about resource allocation, can the figures be manipulated in ways that are difficult or impossible to detect?[21] It would be easy to improve a hospital's apparent results. Episode inflation could increase the denominator while the numerator remains the same. There is considerable scope for this, given the loose definition of a finished consultant episode.[22] There is clearly a need to move away from information systems based on finished consultant episodes, although the government is unwilling to do so as it would undermine some of its claims for the apparent success of the NHS reforms.[23]

The limitations of ICD-9 and the extent to which clinical judgment can influence the allocation of diagnostic codes means that it is relatively easy to move a substantial number of patients from one diagnostic category to another. The limitations of severity systems using routine data to identify true differences in severity suggest that it would be advantageous to avoid treating patients who are seriously ill. Finally, the lack of complete data for most providers means that there is considerable scope for misplacing the case notes for those patients who die, thus reducing the chances of them being entered into the data set.

If mortality league tables become a reality, it is most likely that provider behaviour will change to incorporate some or all of these tactics. There is clear evidence from the United States that the introduction of prospective payment led to substantial changes in diagnostic coding, to the advantage of providers.[24] There is also evidence that the introduction of the finished consultant episodes in the United Kingdom led to an increase in the capture of episodes, resulting in an apparent increase in activity.[25] In the education sector, there is growing evidence that schools judged on A-level success rates are refusing less able pupils entry to the exams.

Interpretation

If it is possible to overcome all of the problems that have been identified, and the evidence suggests that this is not the case, what should be done with the results? There are many situations in which it is known that the outcome is different in one situation than in another but it is less clear how to interpret the difference. For example, there is good evidence that outcome correlates well with the volume of procedures undertaken for some interventions.

There are two possible reasons for this. It could be because practice makes perfect – the more you do the better you become. Alternatively, it could be due to selective referral, with those who are best at doing something being sent more patients; or it could be due to a combination of both reasons.[26]

A correct interpretation is clearly important because of the implications for policy on such things as regionalisation of hospitals, but findings from routine data are inconsistent. Death rates, as a measure of outcome, are especially limited because death is not always an adverse event; for people with terminal disease, a peaceful and pain free death is a good outcome.

Conclusion

It has been argued that publication of league tables will provide the stimulus to overcome the difficulties but this suggests ignorance of the methodological issues involved. Unfortunately, given the necessity to equalise the possession of information across the purchaser-provider split if the market is to work, and given the record in other sectors of public policy, these problems are unlikely to prevent the publication of league tables. If they are to be published several steps must be taken if they are to have any credibility. These include: the development of a mechanism for severity adjustment specific to Britain; replacement of the finished consultant episode with an improved measure; expansion of record linkage programmes; a major investment in improved data quality; and a process of information audit, with independent external validation of routine data and medical records. Some problems, such as the issue of small numbers, cannot be overcome – and even with comprehensive (and thus extremely expensive) data audit it will not be possible to prevent every case of data manipulation because of the intrinsic uncertainty associated with many definitions. Finally, it is still far from clear that observed differences in mortality actually reflect differences in quality of care.

In summary, some of the technical problems facing those who wish to publish league tables of death rates could be overcome, but at considerable expense. Some, such as independent data audit, may now be necessary because of the changes in the way data are being collected in some hospitals with the effect of maximising income. It is not, however, clear that such an investment would improve the quality of care; through the opportunity cost involved and by creating perverse incentives, it might actually reduce the quality of care. As one American commentator has noted, "the pitfalls of using coded data are generally acknowledged and then thoughtfully ignored."[27] This is not an argument for ignoring differences in death rates. Rather, it suggests that their study should take place in a framework of collaboration between purchaser and provider, and not one of confrontation.

The work on which this paper is based was funded by North West Thames Regional Health Authority. We are grateful to Alison Frater, Trevor Sheldon, and Colin Sanderson for helpful comments at various stages in the work.

1 Laurence J. Patients pay with their lives in operation "lottery". The *Times*. April 27 1993: 1, col 1.

2 Alemi F, Rice J, Hankins R. Predicting in-hospital survival of myocardial infarction: a comparative study of severity issues. *Med Care* 1990; 28: 762–75.

3 McKee M, Hunter D. *Mortality league tables. A comparison of hospital death rates in North West Thames region.* London: London School of Hygiene and Tropical Medicine, 1994.

4 Gonnella JS, Hornbrook MC, Louis DZ. Staging of disease: a case-mix measurement. *JAMA* 1984; 251: 637–44.

5 Hartz AJ, Kuhn EM, Pryor DB, Krakauer H, Young M, Heudebert G, *et al*. Mortality after coronary angioplasty and coronary bypass surgery (the national Medicare experience). *Am J Cardiol* 1992; 1: 179–85.

6 RITA study group. Coronary angioplasty versus coronary artery bypass surgery: the Randomised Intervention Treatment of Angina (RITA) trial. *Lancet* 1993; 341: 573–80.

7 Roos NP, Ramsey EW. A population based study of prostatectomy: outcomes associated with different surgical approaches. *J Urol* 1987; 137: 1184–8.

8 Malenka DJ, Roos N, Fisher ES, McLerran D, Whaley FS, Barry MJ, *et al*. Further study of the increased mortality following transurethral prostatectomy: a chart based analysis. *J Urol* 1990; 144: 224–8.

9 Andersen TF, Bronnum-Hansen H, Sejr T, Reopstorff C. Elevated mortality following transurethral resection of the prostate for benign prostatic hypertrophy: but why? *Med Care* 1990; 28: 870–81.

10 Concato J, Horwitz RI, Feinstein AR, Elmore JG, Schiff SF. Problems of comorbidity in mortality after prostatectomy. *JAMA* 1992; 267: 1077–82.

11 Knaus WA, Draper EA, Wagner DP, Zimmerman JE. APACHE II: A severity of disease classification system. *Crit Care Med* 1985; 13: 818–29.

12 Sellar C, Goldacre MJ, Hawton K. Reliability of routine hospital data on poisoning as measures of deliberate self-poisoning in adolescents. *J Epidemiol Community Health* 1990; 44: 313–5.

13 Iezzoni LI. Using administrative diagnostic data to assess the quality of hospital care: pitfalls and potential of ICD-9CM. *Int J Technol Assess Health Care* 1990; 6: 272–81.

14 Abrams P. New words for old: urinary tract symptoms for "prostatism". *BMJ* 1994; 308: 929–10.

15 Vickers N, Pollock A. Incompleteness and retrieval of case notes in a case note audit of colorectal cancer. *Quality in Health Care* 1993; 2: 170–4.

16 Gulliford MC, Petruckevitch A, Burney PG. Hospital case notes and medical audit: evaluation of non-response. *BMJ* 1991; 302: 1128–9.

17 Jencks SF, Williams DK, Kay T. Assessing hospital associated deaths from discharge data: the role of length of stay and comorbidities. *JAMA* 1988; 260: 2240–6.

18 Breslow NE, Day NE. *Statistical methods in cancer research*. Vol 2. *The design and analysis of cohort studies*. Lyons: International Association for Research on Cancer, 1987.
19 Palmer CR. Probability of recurrence of extreme data: an aid to decision making. *Lancet* 1993; **342**: 845–7.
20 Park RE, Brook RH, Kosekoff J, Keesey J, Rubenstein L, Keeler E, et al. Explaining variations in hospital death rates: randomness, severity of illness and quality of care. *JAMA* 1990; **264**: 484–90.
21 Dicing with death rates [editorial]. *Lancet* 1993; **341**: 1183–4.
22 Clarke A, McKee M. The consultant episode: an unhelpful measure. *BMJ* 1992; **305**: 1307–8.
23 Mawhinney B. Hansard. 14 January 1993, col 806.
24 Cohen BB, Pokras R, Meads MS, Krushat WM. How will diagnosis-related groups affect epidemiological research? *Am J Epidemiol* 1987; **126**: 1–9.
25 Clarke A, Tinsley P. Completed consultant episodes and hospital discharge. *BMJ* 1992; **304**: 990.
26 Black NA, Johnston A. Volume and outcome of hospital care: evidence, explanations and implications. *Health Serv Management Rev* 1990; **3**: 108–14.
27 Safran C. Using routinely collected data for clinical research. *Stat Med* 1991; **10**: 559–64.

12 Dicing with death rates

H BRENDAN DEVLIN

Death rates are an emotive topic for consultant surgeons and gynaecologists. Death after surgery is so rare nowadays that to the public a death inevitably connotes that something went wrong. The problem with publishing death rates is that they are perceived as the authorities looking for the "bad apples" rather than identifying the good units where high quality work takes place.

Historically, death rates as an outcome measure were called for by Florence Nightingale in 1880; nobody acted on her advice. The father of surgical audit, Ernest Codman, recommended in 1914, after a trip to England, publishing the "end result" of hospital treatment. A variant of this advice was the basis of the "minimum standards" accreditation programme devised for the American College of Surgeons by John Bowman.

Death rates, as elicited and published by Semmelweis in Vienna, greatly influenced the development of safe obstetric care. In surgery the most explicit early example of published death rates influencing practice is in the German literature in the 1890s. Bassini, the professor of surgery in Padua, published his results of hernia operation in 1894; 262 operations with no operative deaths. Billroth, from Vienna, had his results written up and published by his oberartz, Dr Haidenthaller, in 1890; 195 operations with 11 operative deaths. With these death rates, and other outcome measures, Billroth's technique was abandoned and the basis of modern surgery to this day remains Bassini's operation.

Defining the denominator

The definition of the denominator is an enormous problem. Should the whole population of a district be used as the denominator to work out a death rate standardised for age and sex, the district death rate, to give us something similar to a standard mortality rate? Such a district death rate is already published and allows us to make comparisons between districts and, by inference, says something about patient equity.

Or should death rates use as their denominator all the patients admitted to a hospital, the hospital death rate? This is clearly a way of screening out inadequate surgical selection, but a confounding factor is that, in some hospitals, general practitioners have the right to admit unscreened patients directly for surgery. If too many irrelevant cases are admitted, the death rate may be reduced. Hospital death rates, suitably standardised for age and sex, are an attractive comparator of surgical activity – if all the patients admitted with a particular diagnosis are used as the denominator for the death rate, at least we get a complete case mix situation. Surgeons then cannot exclude the highly complex cases from the operating rooms just to get better death rates.

Would it be more realistic to use the more traditional surgical death rate, which uses all the patients operated on by an

---

Death rates and denominators

District death rate
- Uses whole population of district
- Similar to standard mortality rate

Hospital death rate
- Uses all patients admitted to hospital
- Screens out inadequate surgical selection

Surgical death rate
- Uses all patients operated on by an individual surgeon
- Can easily be manipulated to exclude "poor risk" cases.

Avoidable death rate
- Involves a retrospective "peer group" decision on "avoidability"
- Difficult and time consuming to calculate

---

individual surgeon as the denominator? Of course this overlooks the two issues already referred to.

Another useful indicator of competence is the avoidable death rate. This is difficult and time consuming to calculate in surgical and anaesthetic practice. The original CEPOD report did this and showed wide differences between hospitals.[1] But as these data were confidential and anonymised, nobody commented too much. The profession and the public were just bemused.

Low volume operators and case mix

Looking at death rates it is clearly apparent that volume – that is, the number of operations performed per year – influences the outcome of that operation. There is the problem of the occasional operator; an occasional operator doing only one of one type of operation a year and getting one death a year therefore has a death rate of 100%. It is unlikely at present that this will in any way influence local esteem of the operator, who will always be able to plead that was the best possible in the circumstances. The very low volume, and often deadly, operator is a sad reality as our health service is currently structured. Low volume operators in inappropriate settings are hazardous. Both the operator and the unit team are important to good outcomes.[2, 3, 4]

The next problem with death rates is the problem of case mix. To allow any comparisons, death rates must be corrected and adjusted for age and sex, but the severity of the cases operated on clearly has crucial importance in determining the death rate, as has been shown in many studies. Comorbidities often determine the outcome of surgery, as the confidential inquiries into perioperative deaths have repeatedly shown.

Inadequate data

The next problem with death rates in Britain is the problem of the inadequacy of data. Data in the NHS are plentiful but are often incorrect or may be even inadequately analysed. No data on activities, operations, and mortality in the private sector are publicly available.

If death rates are to be calculated routinely, NHS data sets will need to be improved enormously. A unique patient identifier number, routine recording of comorbidity on the last discharge summary, and, above all, guaranteed correctness will only be achieved when consultants assume responsibility for data collection. In death rates we are talking about problems of sample size and correctness; if death rates are to be taken seriously by the public and profession they must be robust and reliable. The confidential inquiries had hoped to produce national mortality rates; the original inquiry working in three NHS regions was able to produce some data and death rates in 1988. Sadly, since those halcyon days the information from the Department of Health and NHS has deteriorated or is just not there. In the inquiries the lack of a unique patient identifier number prevents us tracking any patient through the interstices of the system. Some ear, nose and throat surgeons in tertiary centres performing terminal tracheostomies on patients in intensive care units seem to be lethal: the data do not allow us to identify the surgeons who performed the original surgery which led to transfer to the intensive care unit, and it is clearly wrong to blame the surgeons who perform the terminal tracheostomy for the bad death rates. The definition and recording of operations is also very poor, leading to further difficulties in any inquiry.

Variations in death rates

Death at operation is rare – approximately 0.6% of all surgical operations end in death. Nowadays much surgery is done for disability or pain or distress rather than to prevent death. Even so, there are big variations in death rates between districts, hospitals, and individual surgeons. In avoidable death rates there are even bigger variations.[1] These warrant an explanation.

To overcome the problems of small numbers, individual consultants' death rates for common operations – and their confidence intervals – could be calculated on a rolling three year basis. These rates should, however, be viewed only as an indicator warranting further investigation before a consultant is pronounced incompetent. We must investigate and help outlier doctors before we condemn and stigmatise them.

Alternative indicators

Which outcomes, apart from death, are useful in looking at surgical performance? Sepsis rates could be used as an alternative to death rates, but here again there are problems with the definition of sepsis, and sepsis is also rare, usually 1-2% in elective surgery, and even then is no more than a nuisance to the patients. Sepsis causing severe problems is rare, apart from when prostheses are introduced.

Recurrence after surgery, be it recurrence of a tumour or recurrence of a hernia or failure of a prosthesis, is more of a problem in surgery and could be used as a good indicator in surgical league tables.

Patient "(dis)satisfaction" probably is the best of all measures of surgical outcome. A dead patient clearly cannot have any satisfaction – and may be a manifestation of dissatisfaction. Recently when I was talking about death rates and patient satisfaction to a band of surgeons, one surgeon told me that it didn't matter whether the patient was satisfied or not providing they had had "the right operation." A dissatisfied customer is always a failure, and surgeons need to recognise this.

Given better data systems, I think we could work out meaningful death rates quite easily. The biggest problem we face is whether they should be published. Many people think they should be, but equally many surgeons vigorously think otherwise. Many in the health service, doctors and administrators, think that everything should be kept under wraps: as long as we can resist the public pressure for disclosure our present configuration of health services remains secure. The most readily available league tables of consultants, validated annually and scientifically rigorous, are distinction awards. As a start towards the new openness we all need on performance, we could start by publishing these.

1 Buck N, Devlin HB, Lunn JN. *Report of a confidential inquiry into perioperative deaths.* London: Nuffield Provncial Hospitals Trust and the King's Fund, 1987
2 Devlin HB, Professional audit: quality control and keeping up to date. *Baillière's Clinical Anaesthesiology* 1988; 2: 299–324.
3 Wennberg JE, Roos N, Sola L, Schori A, Jaffe R. Use of claims data systems to evaluate health care outcomes: mortality and reoperation following prostactectomy. *JAMA* 1987; 257: 933–6.
4 Emberton M, *et al.* The National Prostatectomy Audit 1992–3. *British Journal of Urology* (In press).

13 The health gain issue

J R ASHTON

In recent years the pace of change in the organisation of health systems has become frenetic and this has been paralleled by the shortening half life of new health related jargon. The term "health gain" appeared sometime in 1990–1 and streaked across the sky leaving a turbulence in its wake and people asking, "What was that concept anyway?"

The term health gain is difficult to pin down, but at its heart is some idea of a focus on outcome rather than input or process. It is worth reminding ourselves that until recently we have had no explicit outcome based objective for the NHS other than the aim of the founding fathers in 1948, that treatment should be equally available to all on the basis of need and that it should be free at the time of use. One consequence of this has been almost half a century of normative planning with the emphasis on resource inputs per thousand populations and little effort to relate inputs to outcomes, certainly on a population basis.

The often circular discussions about "what is health?" have rumbled through the literature since the World Health Organisation's definition of 1948. That definition tried to include social and psychological, as well as physical, perspectives. Subsequent proposals have gradually shaken out to underline the importance of health as a resource for everyday life rather than an end in itself, and the issue of quality of life as opposed to quantity has been increasingly recognised – the limitations of coffin counts as health outcome measures for an aging population are becoming daily more apparent.[1]

One of the sources of weakness in our collective thinking has been the divorce of the epidemiological (population) perspective from the clinical focus on the individual patient. This divorce in policy and practice has been reinforced by the medical schools in their teaching and research. Fortunately the implications of this

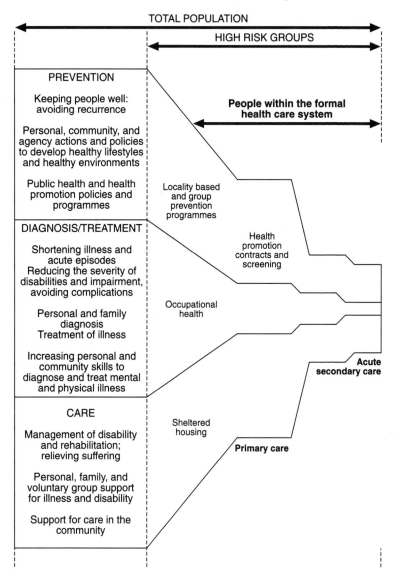

Figure 13.1 Framework for investments relating inputs to outcomes and making roles explicit

have recently begun to be recognised, and the current round of curricular change provides an opportunity for a fresh start.[2-4] In the former Mersey region, the health policy unit has distilled down this debate to provide three explicit objectives for the NHS.

• Keeping people well
• Getting people better
• Looking after people.[5, 6]

In taking Geoffrey Rose's "prevention paradox"[7] into mainstream policy formation the unit has developed a framework for considering how a balanced portfolio of investment might begin to relate inputs to outcomes which maximise health gain in these three areas and which make explicit the role of both alliances for health and the contributions of individuals, families, and other social groups, including employers, to improving the health of the population (figure 13.1). The implications of this are that, on the one hand, a twin track approach of programmes for the population and for high risk groups is necessary; on the other hand, the ethical implications of trade offs between the two of these tracks need to be confronted (figure 13.2).

Sir George Godber has pointed out that "equity in health care would not be equality; the worst off would need the most"; on the basis of Geoffrey Rose's prevention paradox the uncomfortable conclusion is that there will be greater health gain pro rata from investment in population based programmes than in programmes for those at high risk or whose health is already damaged and among whom deprived people are over-represented (figure 13.3).

To take this to its logical conclusion, we may wish to give priority to population based programmes for planned parenthood and giving children a good start in life – free from poverty and equipped with adequate education and full nutrition – so that they reach adulthood with a minimum amount of baggage to prejudice their future health.

In a more general way, with our commitment to getting away from bodies in beds as an index of health service performance clearly in mind, we might wish to underline the contribution to the health gain of populations of horizontal rather than vertical interventions – that is, interventions that affect whole populations and prevent multiple conditions rather than magic bullets for high risk or diseased groups for single conditions. Historical examples

123

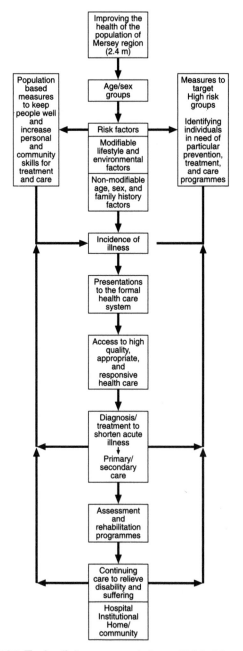

Figure 13.2 Trade offs between population and high risk approaches

124

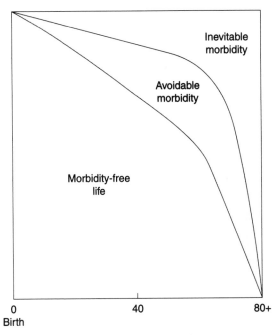

Figure 13.3 The scope for compressing the morbidity curve and adding life to years

of fundamentally important horizontal interventions include the provision of safe food, water, and sanitation. Today's examples would be planned parenthood, safer sex, and tobacco free and safe environments. Poverty and ignorance unite the past with the present and remain a fundamental challenge.

Towards a balanced portfolio of investment for health gain

With these ideas in mind a rational approach to a balanced portfolio of investment would begin with a needs assessment based on an understanding of the structure and distribution of the population, the patterns of health and disease within it, and a sound knowledge of which interventions (hard or soft, technical or social) make what difference (figure 13.4).

It would move on to examine critically which things are worth doing in terms of their levels of need within the population and

125

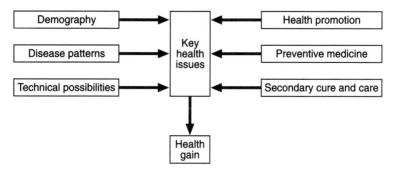

Figure 13.4 Assessing health need and achieving health gain

the increasing health gains for investment made – focusing investment on the stars, disinvesting from the dogs and giving serious consideration to how to maximise the health gains from cash cows and those programmes over which there is a question mark (figure 13.5). We might finish up with a menu similar to that in the boxes.

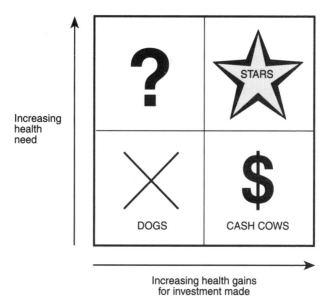

Figure 13.5 Health programme portfolio management

Best bets for health gain

Primary interventions/health promotion:

Tobacco free environment
Moderate alcohol use
More exercise
Planned parenthood
Safe sex
Immunisation programmes
Accident prevention
Environmental (ecological) issues

Secondary interventions:

Good primary care in poor areas
Good screening and case finding services (hypertension, cervical
    cancer, breast cancer, etc)
Mental health promotion
Chronic disease care

Tertiary interventions:

Clinical protocols
Peer audit
External monitoring

A mechanism for planning for health gain

The agenda for future health is broad – the advice that is
needed for it is a world apart from that traditionally provided to
health authorities by medical advisory committees with their
narrow disciplinary and institutional perspective and their wish
lists with no evidence of the population outcomes that would
result. This is not to belittle the relevance or importance of
technical advice but rather to argue the necessity for it to be set in
a context which is social and cultural, economic and scientific, and
ethical. It must also consider the balance of health promotion,
primary, secondary, and tertiary interventions. One approach to
this problem was piloted in 1992 by Yorkshire Health, the Eastern
Health and Social Services Board, and Mersey Regional Health

Authority, focusing on three issues – coronary heart disease, antenatal screening for congenital malformations, and teenage planned parenthood. In each case the relevant critical biological, epidemiological, health economic, and outcomes data were brought together as far as these were available and considered in a day long workshop which included biologists, clinicians, public health staff, health economists, managers, and an ethicist. A workshop format which allowed for presentations of positions and rigorous interrogation resulted in moves towards consensus about a balanced approach to commissioning and resource allocation which might not have been anticipated before the workshop.

1 Ashton J, Seymour H. *The new public health*. Milton Keynes: Open University Press, 1988.
2 White KL. *Healing the schism; epidemiology, medicine and the public's health*. New York: Springer Verlag, 1991.
3 White KL, Connelly JE, eds. *The medical school's mission and the population's health*. New York: Springer Verlag, 1992.
4 Ashton J. Institutes of public health and medical schools: grasping defeat from the jaws of victory? *J Epidemiol Community Health* 1993; 47 (3): 165–8.
5 Mersey Regional Health Authority. *Strategic framework*. Liverpool: MRHA, 1993.
6 Mersey Regional Health Authority. *Strategic Statement*. Liverpool: MHRA, 1994.
7 Rose G. *The strategy of preventive medicine*. Oxford: Oxford Medical Publications, 1992.
8 Godber G. Medical Officers of Health and Health Services. *Community Medicine* 1986; 8: 1–14.
9 Eastern Health and Social Services Board, Mersey Regional Health Authority, Yorkshire Health. *Health gain. Health gain seminars summary*. Liverpool: Liverpool Public Health Observatory, Department of Public Health, University of Liverpool, 1992.

14 Casemix: isoneed, iso-outcome, and health benefit groups

HUGH SANDERSON

The IM and T strategy

The NHS information management and technology strategy provides a vision for the development of information to support the delivery of care. The vision essentially sees the development of information technology to support the whole process of patient care, including the patient record. Ultimately, it is aimed at delivering patient based systems which capture clinical information at the point of care, hold information that can be used for patient care, and needs to be entered only once. These systems will be capable of supporting both better clinical care, and better management decisions.

Using clinical terms to describe patients and clinical care

To support these clinical records, a suitable set of terms must be developed. These terms can be used by all health care professionals to record everything that they need to record about an individual patient and the process of care that the patient receives. This thesaurus of terms has been the subject of the Clinical Terms Project and the companion Nursing and Professions Allied to Medicine Terms Projects. These projects are delivering the core and qualifying terms required to capture the clinical record in very considerable detail.

When completed, these projects will have specified several hundred thousand discrete terms, and the combinations of terms for each individual patient will be very complex indeed. It will therefore be necessary to ensure that ways of combining the terms into meaningful groups are developed and made available for analysis, to ensure that data fed in can be extracted again. This is similar to the concept of executive information systems, where the raw data at the bottom of the pyramid, which are useful for tactical and local decisions, need to be aggregated to be useful for managers at a higher level, who need to make strategic decisions. Using a different analogy, we can envisage the large wheel of data collection, which needs to drive the equally large wheel of management and clinical decisions, but requiring a small but crucial cog (of patient groupings) to enable the data to drive the decisions.

These aggregations to support comparison are based around two key concepts:

Groupings of patients with similar conditions, and groupings of similar treatments.

Similar treatment groups are isoresource groupings, but similar condition groups can provide both isoneed groups and iso-outcome groups. That is to say, for patients with similar conditions there is a similar expectation of the care that should be provided; and these patients, provided that similar care has been provided, should have a similar outcome. In order to convey this meaning they are labelled health benefit groups.

Potential application of condition groups

The application of isoresource groups is mainly in the area of management of resources, whether this is within a provider unit, to manage the internal resource, or to provide information to help resource allocation by a purchaser to provider. This requires groupings of treatments that can be readily costed and that enable providers to recover the fair costs of treatment.

Isoneed and iso-outcome groups, on the other hand, are of

much more use to the purchaser. Isoneed groups could be used to enable a purchaser to translate the epidemiological information about the population into an assessment of the care required. Iso-outcome groups will enable purchasers and providers to examine the outcomes achieved and compare them to the outcomes expected.

These two concepts can be combined very simplistically by considering the condition and the treatment package within a two dimensional matrix. In this way we can consider the types of conditions (grouped by severity, and capable of predicting the appropriate treatment response) against the treatment packages that may be appropriate for several different conditions. The combination of the condition and the treatment provides iso-outcome groups in which a particular level of outcome is expected for that severity of condition and that package of care.

In the example of this model (figure 14.1) a proportion of patients with condition A receive treatment D; similarly, this treatment is appropriate for condition B. Treatment B, too, is appropriate for condition B. The actual specification of the percentages of cases within each cell of the example has not been included, since this is an issue which should be discussed and negotiated on the basis of good quality health services research. In principle, however, the approach provides a framework for systematising the use of patient based information about the epidemiology of conditions in the population and the use of health service resources.

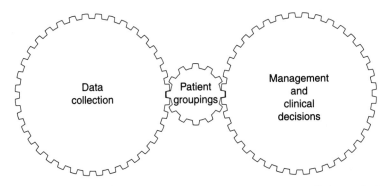

Figure 14.1 For the large wheel of data collection to drive the equally large wheel of management and clinical decisions, a small but crucial cog – of patient groupings – is needed

Constraints on developing condition groups

If we are to develop groupings of similar conditions with similar needs and similar outcomes, then the groupings will need to be based around both the "condition/diagnosis" and the severity of the condition. This raises some issues that need to be considered, and there has been considerable research and literature in the area, much of which comes from the United States.[1]

Definitions of severity

Most of the work undertaken on such groupings has been focused on the issue of adjusting risk of adverse outcome, so that the definition of severity is based on increased risk of death or disability. The other main focus has been on defining ways of refining the prediction of resource consumption of diagnosis related groups (DRGs).

Ways of defining severity are therefore based on the outcome of interest (death, organ failure, disability, length of stay, etc). For predicting the needs of care, these definitions of severity may not be sufficient, as issues of the expected benefit of particular interventions may be important. In addition, the time scale of the expected outcome may differ between specialties, since intensive care scores with a focus on survival over a few days may be quite different from cancer scores with a focus on five year survival.

Generic versus disease specific approaches

Much work has been carried out on disease specific and generic approaches to rating severity and risk of adverse outcome. Both of these approaches seem to be important – for example, TNM stage in malignant disease is important in predicting the requirements for both care and outcome, but a global performance scale is also important in assessing the likely response to treatment and the best therapeutic options. Similarly, a review of methods has suggested that "a productive approach for risk adjusting in hospital mortality figures may involve adding a small subset of disease specific variables to a core group of general physiological findings."[2]

Endogenous versus exogenous

It may seem obvious, when grouping patients with similar needs, that the grouping should be based on the characteristics of the patient (endogenous) rather than on external treatment factors (exogenous). However, some grouping systems include treatment variables and this reduces their suitability for predicting need or outcomes.

Data requirements

The data required for allocating patients into similar need and outcome groups may consist of both disease specific and generic variables. In general, these data go beyond the type of data that is currently collected by routine information systems.

Attempts have been made in Disease Staging to use diagnostic codes to classify severity levels within specific conditions; these predict the mortality risk. Other systems, however, have concentrated on using more clinical data, and up to now this has required specific data collection from patient notes. This has obviously been very expensive to do routinely with paper based records, but in a future of electronic clinical records in which data have captured as Read terms this kind of constraint may be expected to disappear.

Timing

In predicting the needs for care and the likely outcome of care, the timing of data collection and of making the prediction, in relation to the start of the illness or treatment, is crucial. Some systems attempt to provide predictions by using discharge diagnoses; others insist on the collection of data within a specified period of the start of the treatment episode. These issues may become less of a constraint with the introduction of electronic clinical records, but until then the capture of information at other points in time will be expensive.

The National Casemix Office's development programme

The work of the National Casemix Office is based on trying to meet short and long term requirements.

In the short term, there is a need for making use of the data that is currently available routinely. This is likely to be based on discharge diagnosis, in terms of the International Classification of Diseases and have all the limitations of ICD for this purpose.

However, these codes may provide some useful ways of examining the data. The most useful model for this kind of grouping system is Disease Staging, and it may be that much of the logic of this approach can be used.

In the longer term, the greater availability of data about the patient will provide opportunities to move towards the more extensive models of severity scoring, such as MedisGrps, Computerised Severity Index, APACHE, etc. Elements of these are likely to be incorporated into groupings based upon the detailed information held in a Read coded data set. At this stage it should be possible to construct much more clinically sensitive and accurate groups; however, the statistical data to support the grouping definitions may not be available for many years.

These grouping methods will be applied within the purchasing framework, for purchasers to make use of epidemiological data to assess the purchasing needs of their population, and will also be used by providers and purchasers for clinical data, combining the condition group and treatment group as an audit tool to assess the relation between the actual and expected outcome.

1 Orchard C. Comparing healthcare outcomes. *BMJ* 1994; **309**: 1493–6.
2 Iezzoni L, *et al.* Predicting in hospital mortality. A comparison of severity measurement approaches. *Med Care* 1993; **30**: 347–59.

15 Outcomes and general practice

MIKE PRINGLE

Despite nearly three decades of devotion to Donebedian's triad of structure, process, and outcome – a mantra that has now assumed mystical connotations – primary care has tended to focus on the first two at the expense of the third. It might be thought that structure would be relatively easy to measure. The number of whole time equivalent practice nurses, the floor area of the medical centre, the distance to secondary care services – all these structures can be defined and measured. However, it might be argued that the number of patients registered and their health status and needs are also part of the structure. This is where artificial divisions become difficult.

If a practice has a high proportion of women who have not had cervical cytology, this could be said to be a component of the health needs profile of the practice and to reflect the structure in which the practice operates. It might just as validly be supposed that the low rate reflects the preceding process of care and is a measure of that process. A case could, however, be made for regarding the low uptake of cervical cytology as a proxy for outcome: a low uptake should lead to later diagnosis of, and a higher mortality from, cervical cancer. This interpretation of a quasi-outcome role is compatible with the introduction of target payments for cervical cytology, and is comparable to the use of control of glycaemia as proxy for outcomes in diabetes or blood pressure for hypertension.

Any superficial examination of the triad shows that its apparent certainty conceals a wealth of inconsistency and blurring. This is

135

as true of the outcomes category as of the others, and in this paper I will try to find a pragmatic route towards a definition of outcomes in general practice and their measurement.

Traditional outcome measures

There is an attraction to those outcomes which can be identified, categorised, and counted with accuracy. The most obvious of these is death. My practice of 5600 patients had 81 deaths in 1991-2 and 77 in 1992-3. Of those in 1992-3, 20 (26%) were due to cancer, 8 (10%) to stroke, 10 (13%) to respiratory disease, 22 (29%) to ischaemic heart disease, 4 (5%) to old age, and 13 (17%) to other causes. It is apparent that changes in such small numbers are unlikely to be of use in monitoring changes in the health or the quality of health services for our population.

As an example, what are we to make of the fact that there were 20 deaths from respiratory disease in 1991-2 but only 10 in 1992-3? Even this apparent halving of a death rate just fails to reach statistical significance ($P = 0.09$) due to small numbers, but it would be a dramatic intervention which had such an effect in one year. Of course, we know that most respiratory deaths occur in very old people and are not suitable for, nor amenable to, intervention (none were due to asthma). However, the point is that if an effective intervention were to be applied to, say, cancer then the numbers of patients in a single practice would be too few to reliably demonstrate the effect.

While the reports of regional and district directors of public health continue to emphasise overall mortality, individual practices must look elsewhere.

The Health of the Nation

It still seems surprising that a £30 billion enterprise could have existed for 40 years and could have been radically reorganised without its main outcomes being defined. Not until the Health of the Nation initiative was published did we have clear priority areas and targets within them. Another surprise was to realise how great were the expectations from primary care.

Each area and target was chosen to meet three main criteria. The first was that it had to represent a major health issue;

secondly, it must be amenable to effective intervention; and, lastly, it must be capable of being monitored. The last of these stipulations meant that many of the first set of targets were mortality based, and others were based on episodically collected population health data. In the future the data to monitor these targets should be available in primary care, and new targets can be devised that rely on the rich possibilities of general practice databases.

However, the real challenge for primary care lies in the "effective intervention" clause. If the targets on heart disease, stroke, suicide, unplanned pregnancies, and sexually transmitted diseases are to be met, and if smoking, alcohol, diet, and sexual habits are to change, then primary care must inevitably be the arena for action. The Health of the Nation can be seen, therefore, as having set the outcome measures for general practices as a whole. Yet these targets are difficult to assess in individual practices. My practice provides examples (tables 15.1 and 15.2).

The Health of the Nation target for smoking, for example, is to have no more than 20% of adults smoking by the year 2000. Our female population is very nearly there, unless the one fifth not recorded are predominantly smokers. Does this reflect good care on behalf of the practice, or is it a reflection on the middle class nature of our practice area? I suspect it is the latter. Should we, perhaps, now relax about smoking and concentrate on obesity, where the Health of the Nation target is for 8% of women to have a body mass index over 29? As a practice team we feel powerless in the face of the affluence driven explosion of obesity.

We are already under the targets for both men and women for alcohol consumption. Does this reflect again our middle class clientele or, more realistically, reflect the fact that our patients understand the benefits of being economical with the truth? I

Table 15.1 Lifestyle variables recorded on practice computer

Variable	No (%) of adult patients (n = 4131)
Smoking status	3383 (81.9)
Alcohol intake	3354 (81.2)
Blood pressure	3350 (81.1)
Body mass index	2809 (68.0)

Table 15.2 Patients with high lifestyle values recorded on practice computer

	No (%) of adult patients		
	All	Men	Women
Current smoker	810 (24.1)	414 (28.3)	396 (20.6)
Alcohol > recommended level	349 (10.4)	249 (16.8)	100 (5.3)
Systolic blood pressure > 160	399 (11.9)	177 (12.0)	222 (11.8)
Diastolic blood pressure > 95	291 (8.7)	141 (9.6)	150 (7.9)
Body mass index > 29	354 (12.6)	136 (11.5)	218 (18.6)

suspect that many lead blameless lives for a week before their well person checks in order to be able to offer exemplary drinking habits, only to resort to the pub after their check to make up for lost time.

As useful as the Health of the Nation targets are for the country and for large populations, it can be seen that each practice needs to assess its performance and set itself new targets. These might be lower or higher than the Health of the Nation ones, but they should be realistic while being challenging.

Towards a definition of outcomes in primary care

The three Health of the Nation criteria for targets are valid in primary care, but they need to be defined within the primary care setting. Asthma, for example, is a very important disease which is amenable to intervention and which can be monitored in primary care. While mortality is, thankfully, too infrequent to be useful as a measure, many aspects of the process of care and clinical control can be used.

A practice might, for example, measure patients' satisfaction with their care, including emergency advice, or it might monitor compliance. It might set standards for acute care (indications and regimen for use of oral steroids; the use and monitoring of nebulisers; the use of inhaled steroid before the crisis) or for continuing care. Peak flow readings can be recorded and monitored; the giving of a home peak flow meter and instructions on when to respond to falls in lung function can be audited; the prescribing of prophylactic drugs can be recorded.

All these measures are proxies for outcomes, but the most

important outcomes are neglected at the qualitative level in general practice. We do not routinely measure quality of life; activity levels, social functioning, psychological distress, patients' perception of their asthma, and objective symptom control. These are all difficult and easy standardised tools are not yet available, but most practitioners rate them highly as quality markers. If asked why they started an asthma clinic, most doctors talk at first about emergencies and their avoidance. However, they quickly move on to the real issue of primary care – quality of life and minimising symptoms.

This problem is not unique to asthma. Almost all care offered in primary care is geared not to avoiding death but to reducing morbidity, which includes the morbidity of lowered wellbeing. We need to accept measures of clinical control and other proxies for clinical outcome, and augment them with real, objective measures of wellbeing – not inventories that take half an hour, an IQ of 150, and a pair of spectacles to complete, but brief discriminating questions, such as the CAGE questions, that can be repeated often and, if necessary, administered by receptionists.

It has to be asked, however, whether any table of numbers or quality of life measures can ever measure quality of care as it is understood in the 200 million or so consultations in primary care every year. For example, what if I show that the mean glycosylated haemoglobin of my patients with diabetes has fallen in the past few years and that more patients report greater wellbeing – but a thirty year old patient has been registered blind with diabetic retinopathy? Supposing I show, as I have done, that we have a recorded blood pressure in over 80% of our adults, but a 52 year old has a stroke and there is no recorded blood pressure in his medical record? You might wish to ask quite a few questions before commending me on "improved outcomes."

By emphasising cohorts and the meaningfully measurable we must not forget the important. Faced with this imperative, my practice has decided to adopt another, complementary, approach to outcomes. Every month we meet and discuss significant events in the life of the practice. These include every stroke, myocardial infarction, new diagnosis of cancer, suicide attempt, unplanned pregnancy, patient complaint, patient leaving the practice without changing address, visit accepted but not done, patient waiting over 30 minutes after the appointment time – and so on. Some of these are not outcomes in our sense, but they are all outcomes of the clinical and administrative commitment of the practice. We look at each of these events and ask, was everything possible done that should have been done?

The discussion of a significant event may, and often does, result in congratulations. The care was of the highest level. Sometimes, however, the case reveals a lapse in our care; if this is a systematic lapse we put it right. Sometimes we don't know how to react to the case, and we organise a conventional audit to establish the general situation. However, the main verity remains – we look to the experience of individual cases to reflect our inner construct of outcome. This construct has less to do with population targets and more to do with the quality of personal caring that can make the world of difference between different "outcomes" (in the widest sense).

Conclusions

I believe that the current public health/epidemiology model of outcomes is of limited application in primary care. Mortality cannot realistically be monitored at the practice level, and local variations often make national standards seem inappropriate. The conventional gold standards for clinical control and morbidity which have been developed in secondary care are useful (where would we be without the glycosylated haemoglobin and blood pressure?) but cannot tell the whole story.

There is a need for outcome measures that reflect the "quality" part of "quality of care"; measures of wellbeing and functioning in the face of the tides of life. We all grow old, but we all pray to grow old gracefully and with dignity. Only when we can measure the concepts embodied in these sentiments can we truly measure outcomes. One mechanism for monitoring outcomes may be to audit significant events, but it needs to be combined with a flexible and comprehensive population approach.

16 View from NHS management

PAMELA CHARLWOOD

Once upon a time, quality and effectiveness in clinical practice was regarded by many people as a no go area for NHS managers. Now, it is explicitly the business of management. At their peril, however, will chief executives attempt to go it alone, and the prudent chief executive will work with clinical colleagues such as the medical director, clinical director, or director of public health. However, chief executives are increasingly coming to understand that the responsibility for delivering effective services is actually theirs. This was well illustrated recently when the Health Select Committee took to task the chief executive of the NHS in Scotland for apparently failing to ensure that information on effectiveness in clinical practice was known to clinicians and implemented.

Why has the world changed so much in this respect? Is it because managers enjoy telling doctors and other clinicians what to do? Is it because managers are obsessed by the financial bottom line, like their caricatures in the television dramas? I believe it is for the most part because most of the NHS managers I know have a genuine concern for the quality and effectiveness of services provided for patients, and this arises every bit as much from their concern about what it feels like for the patient as from concern for value for money.

We are all aware of the imbalance between the knowledge that is available about effective treatment and the patchy implementation of this. Managers are not paragons in this respect in their own field, but they, at least, are attuned to the fact that when they are told to do something they turn to it with all seriousness. It is beginning to be made clear to them that this approach applies not only to balancing the books and meeting national targets in areas such as waiting times but also to ensuring that knowledge about effectiveness is applied both to purchasing decisions and to provider practice.

When I started to write this, I intended to divide the next section between the benefit of applying knowledge about effective outcomes from the patient's point of view and the benefit in terms of value for money. Unsurprisingly, what I found was that it is virtually impossible to separate the two. The competent management of costs and the achievement of high standards live remarkably close together. In a few cases, we may spend less money because we are ignoring a problem or treating it badly – an example which comes to mind is incontinence – but for the most part, work that is clinically effective is also cost effective. What is more, a lot of this is down to earth, and not necessarily about highly complex and technical issues.

Take the recent report from the chief medical officer about cancer services: survival rates, the appropriate treatment for breast cancer, correct doses of radiotherapy and highly expensive drugs: all of this was presented lucidly and clearly, to be easily understood by lay people, let alone managers and others working within the service. The avoidance, or at least early and effective treatment of pressure sores, is another down to earth example. It was this subject on the agenda of Exeter and North Devon Health Authority which drew record numbers of the public to a meeting of the authority last year. The room could not accommodate all those who were interested in hearing what the health authority was going to do about this basic problem which affected so many elderly people in hospital and in the community. If these issues are of such interest to the public, they must be of importance to managers.

Information on effectiveness

Many other topics are well known both to clinicians and managers: the incidence of myringotomy, removal of tonsils and adenoids, hysterectomy – the arguments and variation in treatment rates across the country are well rehearsed. The chief executive of almost any trust can quote to you the variation in length of stay for lens implant for cataract between their different ophthalmic surgeons; they will range between those surgeons who are approaching perhaps 80% of lens implants as day surgery cases and those who are routinely keeping their patients in hospital for two or even three nights. This variation has little to do with effectiveness of outcome but is a particularly clear example of difference in value for money.

There are many areas of less familiar territory in terms of the research into effectiveness: these areas relate particularly to the less glamorous aspects of clinical practice such as outpatients and primary care. In many cases, information on effectiveness is available but clinicians and managers have been even more reluctant to familiarise themselves with it and change practice as a result. Practice in outpatient clinics is a classic example. Managers – as well as clinicians – have generally been far less excited by outpatient services and, in career terms, a management post in outpatients has never been the route to stardom. So it has been with the commissioning and implementation of research about effectiveness in outpatients. I am reminded particularly of the "different SHO" syndrome: what proportion of repeat appointments are given on a six monthly basis by the senior house officer – who will not be there when the patient reattends? In these circumstances, most senior house officers remain reluctant or feel powerless to discharge a long term patient; so they take the line of least resistance.

A similar story might well be told of many diabetic outpatient clinics if the supervision of junior staff is inadequate: far better to invest the effort in training and supporting a higher number of general practitioners to maintain their patients on a long term basis than have them seen by a series of less than experienced junior doctors, thus freeing up time for those waiting for a first outpatient appointment. I commend the excellent publication of the Health Care Evaluation Unit at the University of Bristol, *Evaluation of Delivery and Use of Outpatient Services*, which now has its place on the desk of trust managers throughout the south west.

Palliative care, the treatment of minor injuries by general practitioners, psychiatric services: these are all areas where information is available but may be passed over as being insufficiently exciting to command attention. Psychiatric services

143

in particular are often felt to be a mystical art rather than a science, with outcomes difficult to measure and the difference in practice between different schools of psychiatry so great that work on effectiveness is not generally applicable. This cannot and must not be so. The money spent on the treatment of schizophrenia is one of the largest areas of spending in the NHS as a whole: surely we cannot fail to be interested in how effective that treatment is? Child and adolescent psychiatry is another example of woeful lack of interest from managers and clinicians other than those clinicians working specifically in that area. And yet what could be a more vital area than the prevention of long term mental instability, self harm, and harm to others? This is a service which in many parts of the country is virtually in crisis, and the approach of purchasers is less than impressive: a prime example of where purchasing decisions should be made on good quality information about outcomes and effectiveness.

I have emphasised all of these practical, down to earth examples in order to encourage managers to believe that the understanding of issues around effectiveness and outcomes is not a rarefied science confined to people working full time in research. It is everybody's business.

Interfaces

As we move on to the practicalities of how to make progress, we encounter a series of interfaces. The first interface is that between primary and secondary care: clinicians working in primary care know a lot about the variation and quality of practice of their colleagues in secondary care, and vice versa; the flow of information across the divide is absolutely essential. I am not one of the purists who believe that research and development and the sophisticated programme of work on effectiveness and outcomes are totally separate from audit: I believe that the areas are firmly and closely interlinked and we would gain much by drawing together far more closely the audit carried out substantially separately in primary and secondary care. Indeed, this was one of the requirements attached to the allocation of the money earmarked for clinical audit in the South West region last year.

Secondly, we have the interface between managers and

clinicians. How should we educate managers, and how should they then work with and seek to influence their clinical colleagues? Indeed, the reverse might apply as frustrated clinicians seek to achieve change sometimes to find it blocked by managerial lack of interest. The first step is continually to present this as a shared agenda and a joint responsibility. All the work that I have been involved in has been approached on this basis and has been the more effective as a result.

Some three years ago Michael Peckham, the Institute of Health Services Management, and the Management Advisory Service held a two day multidisciplinary workshop on health technology assessments. The discussion was broadly based, interpreting health technology in the widest sense and drawing on experience far beyond the United Kingdom. The report which followed from the workshop was a valuable early contribution to raising the awareness of managers that health technology assessment was firmly their business. The institute's seminars, Medicine for Managers, are now in their seventh year, with some thousand managers attending the seminars each year. The programme is devised in partnership between the Institute and Royal Colleges and similar bodies, and the purpose is to provide a briefing for non-clinical staff on current issues and developments in different branches of medicine and clinical practice. It has been particularly interesting in recent years to see these seminars attended by both purchasers and providers, approaching the issues in slightly different but complementary ways.

This interface between purchaser and provider is my third and final area. It is for me both obvious and essential that purchasers must increasingly seek to make their decisions on the basis of knowledge about outcomes.

Moving forward

Within the purchasing organisation, the director of public health should take a lead on quality and effectiveness in clinical practice but should not be so exclusively "the specialist" on outcomes that it is not felt to be anyone else's business or responsibility. It has to be the basis of the entire organisation and its raison d'être. Moreover, the purchaser is unlikely to make consistently sensible and informed decisions if there is not a

145

meeting of minds between purchaser and provider. Among the clinical staff in many if not most trusts will be authors of and contributors to the various studies on effectiveness that purchasers will wish to be using in their discussions with providers. Nationally available information, such as the Health Effectiveness Bulletins and the increasingly valuable products of the regional research and development units, provides the material which purchasers and providers should be discussing together. Indeed, one of the most encouraging areas of development is that of purchasers and providers working together on regional research and development programmes.

More local contacts should be made, and more local use should be made of the information that is available. Medicine for Managers programmes do not have to be held only at national level: the South West region has been looking at setting up "clinical briefings" within the region. The royal colleges need to work increasingly on a multidisciplinary basis at local level to draw in other professional groups, including managers, and to work as effectively in that context to promote good practice as they do in so many respects nationally. Only if it becomes a normal part of the everyday interchange between managers and clinicians locally will we see the development of mutual respect and understanding. This is essential to make far better use of knowledge on effectiveness and outcomes and to see the resulting benefits to patients and to the way in which the NHS uses its money. When I was a regional general manager I put three questions to chief executives of district health authorities. How did you decide what to buy? How will you know if you are getting it? How will you know if it has done anything good? If we can answer these three questions we will be doing well.

17 Measuring mental health outcomes: a perspective from the Royal College of Psychiatrists

JOHN WING

Until recently there have been few relevant laboratory or radiological methods for investigating the major mental illnesses in order to estimate the severity of the underlying processes and thus help to determine outcomes. Perhaps because of this, substantial progress has been made in the measurement of subjective symptoms and behavioural signs. For example, the Present State Examination[1,2] is now in its 10th edition. Algorithms for chapter F of the 10th edition of the International Classification of Diseases have been specified and are used with such instruments to provide reliable diagnoses.[3] Techniques have been devised to measure psychological and social functioning, and computerised methods for collecting clinical and administrative information are in routine use in some health districts.[4] This long tradition has proved invaluable also for measuring outcomes.

Collecting data

The two main aims of outcome research are to facilitate improvements in clinical care (the "clinical audit function") and to provide high quality data to guide public health and purchasing decisions. These two aims are also those of health information

147

systems in general. In other words, collecting data on outcomes should be part of the overall system of health care recording. At the moment, there are two, usually quite separate, perspectives: "bottom up" clinical data, much of it in handwritten records, and "top down" administrative data such as the Körner data set. An opportunity to move forward along both perspectives has been presented by the government's first mental Health of the Nation outcome target: to "improve significantly the health and social functioning of mentally ill people."[5]

The College Research Unit has been commissioned to construct a set of scales simple enough to be used to measure clinical outcomes in routine NHS practice, and also to be incorporated into contracts between purchasers and providers. What we have to do is to measure three apparent imponderables: "mental illness," "health and social functioning," and "significant improvement." However, the background of research and knowledge already accumulated provides a secure platform on which to build.

Before I describe our approach to the problem it will be useful to set out the research strategy into which the outcomes study fits (see box 1). This strategy covers the information needed both for

---

Box 1 – The College Research Unit's research strategy for mental health audit and informatics

1 Preparation of audit guidelines
2 Monitoring audit guidelines
   • Application of electroconvulsive therapy
   • Acute admissions in two health districts
   • Audit of new long stay accommodation
   • Clinical standards of services for schizophrenia
3 SCAN: Schedules for Clinical Assessment in Neuropsychiatry
   • Differential definitions for symptoms and signs
   • Standardisation of clinical interviewing
   • Algorithms for ICD-9, ICD-10, DSM-III-R, DSM-IV
4 Measurement of functional disability
5 Health of the Nation Outcome Scales (HoNOS)
6 Clinical needs assessment
7 Prediction of need in districts
8 Clinical terms project (Read codes)
9 Case mix (mental health related groups)
10 Minimum clinical data set for psychiatry
11 Mental health information systems

Box 2 – Principles of the IMG informatics strategy

- Information will be person based
- Data entered on computer once only
- Public health and administrative data derived from systems used by health care professionals
- Information secure and confidential
- Common standards and networking ensure shared communication across the whole NHS

---

bottom up clinical audit functions and for top down administrative and public health functions.[6, 7] Administrative (including contract) data sets and case mix criteria should be aggregated from the data provided by clinicians.[4, 8] Top down policies can then be driven by clinical (joined to public health) imperatives. There is only one public health continuum. This approach we call "epidemiological responsibility."[1]

An identical strategy has been recommended in a recent booklet from the Information Management Group of the NHS Executive (box 2).[9] The reason for the lack of implementation of these excellent principles lies not only with administrators but with clinicians. Neither group has fully understood the gains to be made by using the new technology.[10–12]

Box 3 – Principles of HoNOS

1 Routine completion by member of mental health team
2 Does not specify a form of interview but records a routine assessment of problems
3 Must be simple; information easily collectable
4 Brief: good coverage in 12 key items
5 Each item is discrete, rated only once
6 Changes between ratings measure outcomes
7 Sensitive to change or lack of it
8 Reasonably reliable and compatible with longer scales of good provenance
9 Yields useful output for:
- Clinical purposes
- Management purposes
- Public health purposes
- Minimum mental health data set

When constructed the Health of the Nation Outcome Scales will provide a small, but highly relevant, instrument for collecting standard, good quality information about mental health outcomes throughout the NHS.[13] In Greek, the acronym (óvos) means donkey, and the instrument is meant to be used as a work horse. It is a useful example for illustration since it involves both bottom up and top down perspectives. The principles guiding the design of HoNOS are listed in box 3. Three intensive pilot phases, using successive versions that gradually came to incorporate the common suggestions of users (principally nurses), resulted in the 12 item instrument currently undergoing field trials.

The 12 items are listed in box 4. Items 1-11 have a five point rating scale, each point of which has its own definition. There are four groups, representing behaviour, impairment, subjective symptoms, and social functioning. The final global scale might be used alone, when rated after the full instrument is complete. Data from the trials will be analysed to discover whether this and other types of summary index will be satisfactory for use for case mix and contracts.

Autonomy

The concept of autonomy deserves further mention since it is applicable to any disease or disability, as indeed are most of the principles of HoNOS. Items 1–8 measure the basic mental health

---

Box 4 – Third draft of HoNOS for field trials

First 11 items are rated on 0–4 scale of severity; item 12 rated 0–100.
 1 Aggression
 2 Self harm
 3 Alcohol and drug use
 4 Memory, orientation
 5 Physical illness or handicap
 6 Mood disturbance
 7 Hallucinations, delusions
 8 Other mental problems
 9 Social relationships and network
10 Autonomy: housing and locality
11 Autonomy: employment, recreation, finance
12 Global rating of function

---

problems that bring people into contact with specialist services. Outcomes on these indices are often favourable. But even when basic impairments persist, such as psychomotor slowness or hallucinosis in schizophrenia, it will often be possible to teach patients how to minimise them and also to help arrange the social environment so that overall handicap is minimised in spite of persisting impairments. There is a close analogy with the counselling and aids that people with physical impairments receive. Items 9–11 measure the extent to which the patient is enabled to exercise optimal autonomy in this way. The concept is close to Hopkins' use of the term "quality of life,"[14] but much of the literature on this concept is diffuse, and most of the scales that purport to measure it are inextricably mixed with the measurement of impairment. Autonomy is not about impairment, which should be measured separately and specifically, but about optimising the functioning of disabled people by providing the opportunity to choose options that otherwise would be out of reach because of impairment.

So far, we are reasonably optimistic that the main trials will confirm and extend the statistical analysis of the pilot results. Some practical problems still needing attention are listed in box 5. The issue of enthusiasm is being investigated by comparing the pilot work (mostly with volunteers) with the main trials, where data collection is routine. If the project is successful the scales will become part of ordinary clinical work and should not be an extra burden. Lifting a version of the scales (derived from the full, clinically collected set) into contracts is being given full attention through public health and purchasing departments, which need to understand and adopt the informatics strategy for themselves.

The issue of league tables is a sensitive one. The results of the

---

Box 5 – Practical problems to be solved

- Top down enthusiasm does not guarantee routine bottom up data collection
- Trials mean extra work for raters
- How would scales be used in contracts?
- Use in league tables
- Relation to other innovations in mental health informatics

field trials will probably show differences between districts, which will be presented in the context of socioeconomic indicators such as the Jarman score and unemployment rates.

Conclusion

The HoNOS project illustrates the work necessary to quantify and make available one small part of the knowledge needed to facilitate and audit clinical work. If successful, it can be used to improve public health, purchasing, and managerial functions. Measuring outcomes, even in this simple fashion, is central to all health informatics, and can help to ensure that the top down and bottom up perspectives become part of one continuum.

The work on HoNOS is supported by research and development funding.

1 World Health Organisation. *SCAN: schedules for clinical assessment in neuropsychiatry.* Version 2. Geneva WHO and APPI (in press).
2 Wing JK, Sartorius N, Üstün TB. *Diagnosis and clinical measurement in psychiatry. A reference manual for the SCAN system.* Cambridge: Cambridge University Press (in press).
3 World Health Organisation. *ICD-10 mental and behavioural disorders. Diagnostic criteria for research.* Geneva: WHO, 1992.
4 Lelliott P, Flannigan C, Shanks S. *A review of seven mental health information systems. A functional perspective.* London: Royal College of Psychiatrists, 1993. (Research Unit publication No 1.)
5 Department of Health. *Health of the Nation key area handbook. Mental health.* London: DoH Health Publications Unit, 1993.
6 College Research Unit. Project and reference list. London: Royal College of Psychiatrists, 1994.
7 Lelliott P. The Royal College of Psychiatrists. In: Hopkins A, ed. *Medical audit of the royal colleges and their faculties in the UK.* London: Pareto Consulting, 1994.
8 Anthony P, Elphick M, Lelliott P. Casemix in psychiatry. *Psychiatric Bulletin* 1992; 17: 8–9.
9 Wing JK. Mental health. In: Stevens A, Raftery J (eds). *Health Care Needs Assessment* vol 2, 202–304. Oxford: Radcliffe Medical Press (in press).
10 Information Management Group. *IM&T strategy overview.* Leeds: NHS Management Executive, 1992.
11 NHS Centre for Coding and Classification. *Read codes and the terms projects. A brief guide.* London: Department of Health, 1993.
12 Lelliott P. Making clinical informatics work. *BMJ* 1994; **308**: 802–3.
13 Wing JK, Rix SR. Read codes for the mental health professions. An update. *Psychiatric Bulletin* 1994; **18**: 234–5.
14 College Research Unit. *Health of the Nation outcome scales for field trials.* London: Royal College of Psychiatrists, 1994.
15 Hopkins A. How might measures of quality of life be useful to me as a clinician? In: Hopkins A, ed. *Measures of the quality of life and the uses to which such measures may be put.* London: Royal College of Physicians, 1994: 1–13.

18 Involving the purchaser through clinical guidelines

JEREMY GRIMSHAW

Clinical guidelines are "systematically developed statements to assist practitioner and patient decisions about appropriate health care for specific clinical circumstances."[1] There is increasing interest in the potential contribution of guidelines in the promotion of evidence based practice[2] to improve patient outcome and efficient resource use. Recently, attention has been focused on how guidelines could be used to inform the commissioning process,[3] shifting the emphasis from buying clinical activity to buying quality clinical care.[4] But considerable professional resistance to the introduction of clinical guidelines remains. Some are concerned that guidelines are insensitive to the needs of individual patients and may thus damage patient care;[5] others are concerned about the restriction of clinical freedom, the medicolegal status of guidelines, and the possible adverse effects of guidelines on future research. Furthermore, there remains uncertainty about whether guidelines can change clinical behaviour,[6] and it is recognised that the successful introduction of guidelines will be slow and difficult.[7]

Within the United Kingdom the systematic development and use of clinical guidelines is relatively new, and experimentation will be required to clarify their role. Fortunately there is a substantial scientific literature which should facilitate the introduction of clinical guidelines. However, if guidelines are to be integrated successfully into contracts and their potential benefits are to be maximised it is important that clinicians, purchasers, and providers understand the scientific basis of clinical guidelines. In this paper I will review our scientific understanding of clinical guidelines and discuss how purchasers and providers may use this knowledge when introducing guidelines within contracts.

Do clinical guidelines change medical practice?

There is a common but incorrect perception that little evidence exists about the effectiveness of clinical guidelines in changing clinicians' behaviour: this is because papers are scattered among many generalist and specialist journals. Ian S Russell and I recently undertook a systematic review of rigorous published evaluations of guidelines.[8] We identified 59 studies covering a wide range of clinical activities.[8] Fifty five of the 59 studies identified improvements in the process of medical care following the development, dissemination, and implementation of guidelines, and all but two of the 11 papers that measured the outcome of care reported improvements. We concluded that guidelines can change clinical practice and lead to improved outcome for patients. To achieve this, however, there were two prerequisites. Firstly, guidelines need to be valid in the sense that when they are followed they actually lead to the health gains and costs predicted for them.[9] Secondly, guidelines must be introduced into clinical practice along with appropriate development, dissemination, and implementation strategies to encourage their adoption by clinicians, thus leading to changes in clinical practice.[10]

Validity of clinical guidelines

It is important to ensure that guidelines are rigorously developed, and thus consistent with the available scientific evidence or, in the absence of such evidence, best clinical judgment. If guideline developers fail to overcome the many potential biases inherent in development, the resulting guidelines may recommend ineffective or even dangerous clinical practice.[9] If guidelines are to be valuable to purchasers it is important that they estimate the likely benefits and costs of their recommendations. It is preferable that a cost effectiveness approach is adopted during guideline development.[12] Greater validity is likely to follow from the use of systematic literature reviews, of national or regional guideline development groups including representatives of all key disciplines, and of explicit links between recommendations and scientific evidence (table 18.1).[9] It is important that developers of a guideline provide adequate documentation to allow potential users (purchasers, providers, and clinicians) to appraise critically its validity and make an informed judgment about whether to adopt it in their clinical practice.[13, 14] Fortunately, guidance on guidelines is available; the NHS Executive is likely to disseminate rigorously developed guidelines[3, 15] and several critical appraisal tools are under development (Rob Hayward, Peter Littlejohn, – personal communications).[16]

Changing clinical practice with clinical guidelines

The successful introduction of guidelines depends on many factors, including the clinical context and the methods by which they are developed, disseminated, and implemented. Various strategies have been proposed to ensure that guidelines change clinical practice,[10, 17–19] but many have not been formally evaluated. Our systematic review[8] suggested that guidelines are more likely to change clinical practice if they are developed by a local group, disseminated by specific educational intervention, and implemented with patient specific prompts during the consultation (table 18.2).[10] Local pilot studies will be required to identify appropriate strategies for different British contexts.

National versus local guidelines

There is a potential conflict between the validity and effectiveness of clinical guidelines. National guidelines are more likely to be scientifically valid, but local guidelines are more likely to change medical practice. The Clinical Resource and Audit Group in Scotland has proposed an attractive solution to this conflict. It suggests that central resources should be devoted to the development of national guidelines, which are "general statements of principle (of good practice)," which should be modified to produce local protocols, which are "more detailed developments of these broad principles for local application."[20] The focus of national guidelines development should be towards ensuring validity. The local development of protocols ensures that they are sensitive to contextual and resource issues, and it

Table 18.1 Factors influencing the validity of clinical guidelines[9]

Likelihood of scientific validity	Method of synthesising evidence	Composition of guideline group			Method of developing guidelines
		Proportion of guideline users	Type of guideline group	No of key disciplines represented	
High	Formal meta-analysis Graded systematic review	Low Low	National external Local external	All	Evidence linked guideline development
Medium	Ungraded systematic review Unsystematic review	Medium	Intermediate	Some	Formal consensus development
Low	Expert opinion	High	Internal	One	Informal consensus development

Table 18.2 Factors influencing the successful introduction of guidelines[11]

Relative probability of being effective	Development strategy	Dissemination strategy	Implementation strategy
High	Internal	Specific educational intervention	Patient specific reminder at time of consultation
Above average	Intermediate	Continuing medical education	Patient specific feedback
Below average	External-local	Mailing targeted groups	General feedback
Low	External-national	Publication in professional journal	General reminder of guidelines

encourages a sense of "ownership" in users. Though this distinction between national and local guidelines is useful, the term protocol may not be immediately acceptable to those who associate the term with rigid and inflexible clinical trial protocols.

Role of guidelines in the commissioning process

Guidelines can be used in various ways in the commissioning process. Guidelines can inform needs assessment by identifying areas of suboptimal care. They can be used to identify and promote good clinical practice in both primary and secondary care settings. At the interface of primary and secondary care they can be used to inform the referral process, thus improving appropriateness of referral; to ensure appropriate use of new procedures or services; to inform secondary care after referral to promote effective health care and reduce unnecessary investigations and treatments; to inform discharge of patients from secondary care to shared or general practitioner care; and to develop criteria and standards for clinical audit and monitoring quality of care.

However, there is little experience of the use of guidelines in the commissioning process. If guidelines are to achieve maximum benefit through the commissioning process, it is important that their introduction is an adequately resourced cooperative venture between clinicians, purchasers, and providers. Clinical audit structures should develop expertise to support development,

157

dissemination and implementation of local guidelines. The purchaser's role in this process includes giving priority to areas in which local guidelines should be introduced; sponsoring development of local guidelines; incorporating guidelines into service specification and contracts; supporting providers' activities to disseminate and implement guidelines; and monitoring the quality standards specified in contracts.

Prioritising areas for local guideline introduction

The successful introduction of guidelines within the NHS will require time to identify the most appropriate and effective dissemination and implementation strategies and the best use of multidisciplinary teams.[21] As the number of guidelines that can be assimilated by health care professionals at any one time is likely to be limited, it is important that local activities are coordinated to prioritise areas for guideline introduction and to limit the number of guidelines that professional groups are asked to implement at any one time.

Needs assessment and clinical audit projects will inform local priority setting by identifying areas of suboptimal clinical care. Greater priority should be given to the introduction of guidelines which address important local needs and for which a rigorously developed national guideline is available for modification. Coordination of local guideline activities should be undertaken by a multidisciplinary group (including representatives of purchasers, providers, and clinicians) with expert leadership, access to structured decision making skills, and relevant information.[22]

Developing local guidelines

Local guideline development should be sponsored jointly by purchasers and providers and be endorsed by relevant clinical groups. Local guideline development groups should be multidisciplinary (including representatives of all key disciplines, purchasers and providers). The success of the group will depend on experienced leadership (by someone "whose disinterested position is unquestioned by any of the concerned parties but whose expertise in coordinating groups of health professionals is accepted by all"[23]) and the presence of technical skills in guideline development within the group (possibly by an experienced facilitator). Clinical audit groups are ideally placed to coordinate and resource local guideline development and should develop expertise in leading and facilitating local guideline development groups.

Where possible, local groups should adapt a rigorously developed national guideline. Local guidelines should include more operational detail than national guidelines. Additional tasks for local groups include identification of resource implications of guideline introduction; barriers to guideline introduction; appropriate dissemination and implementation strategies; and identification of monitoring criteria. Once a local guideline has been developed, it should be pretested by users of the guideline to ensure its face validity, clinical applicability, and acceptability.

Guidelines, service specifications, and contracts

Since the NHS reforms, contracts have tended to concentrate more on "volume" and "price" than on clinical quality issues. Thus there is little experience about how guidelines might be incorporated into contracts. The recent NHS Management Executive letter states that guidelines should "form part of local discussions" (between purchasers and providers).[3] Sheldon and Borowitz say that guidelines should be directly incorporated into purchasing protocols.[4] It is unlikely that detailed clinical guidelines will be included within a contract itself. Guidelines, monitoring criteria, and standards are more likely to be identified within the service specification.

Dissemination and implementation of local guidelines

Dissemination and implementation are the key to ensuring guidelines change clinical practice.[10] Though it will be the role of providers and clinicians to identify appropriate strategies for introducing individual guidelines, purchasers should be prepared to provide support for local experimentation in the short term. In general, new guidelines should be disseminated by specific educational initiatives to all staff whose care is targeted by the guideline and reinforced periodically through continuing professional education. In determining appropriate implementation strategies, it is important to identify which health care professionals are involved in the care targeted by the guideline and the context in which that care is provided. It may then be possible to identify methods of prompting the professional to follow the guideline during the consultation (the most powerful implementation strategy). A variety of strategies may be required to ensure the successful introduction of guidelines.

Monitoring standards

Purchasers and providers need to identify *criteria* (based on guidelines) "to assess the appropriateness of specific health care decisions, services, and outcomes" and a desired *standard of performance* (based on these criteria) which can be monitored through the contracting process to ensure that appropriate quality of care is being provided.[9] Purchasers may increase the desired standard year on year until an optimal standard (defined as "the best which conscientious practitioners can achieve under (normal) working conditions with the resources that are available to them"[24]) is obtained. Providers and local audit structures will be responsible for monitoring standards.

Summary

Following the recent NHS reforms, purchasers are being encouraged to introduce clinical guidelines clarifying the roles of primary and secondary care in patient management and promoting effective health care. Guidelines have the potential to change clinical care and improve patient outcomes, but there is little experience in their use in the commissioning process. If guidelines are to achieve maximum benefit through the commissioning process then clinicians, purchasers and providers need to develop skills in assessing guideline validity and choosing appropriate development, dissemination, and implementation strategies. Resources will be required for developing and implementing guidelines. Local experimentation is essential.

I thank Eileen Barnwell, Simon Capewell, and Hamish Wilson for their helpful comments on earlier drafts of this paper, and Sheila Wallace for help with the literature review. The Health Services Research Unit is funded by the Chief Scientist Office of the Scottish Home and Health Department; however, the opinions expressed in this paper are those of the author and not the funding body.

1 Institute of Medicine. *Guidelines for clinical practice: from development to use.* Washington, DC; National Academic Press, 1992.
2 Guyatt G, Rennie D. Users' guides to the medical literature. *JAMA* 1993; 270: 2096–7.

3 NHS Management Executive. *Improving clinical effectiveness.* Leeds: Department of Health, 1993. (EL (93) 115).
4 Sheldon TA, Borowitz M. Changing the measure of quality in the NHS: from purchasing activity to purchasing protocols. *Quality in Health Care* 1993; 3: 149-50.
5 O'Dowd TC, Wilson AD. Set menus and clinical freedom. *BMJ* 1991; 303: 450-2.
6 Guidelines for doctors in the new world. *Lancet* 1992; 339: 1197-8.
7 Delamothe T. Wanted: guidelines that doctors will follow. *BMJ* 1993; 307: 218.
8 Grimshaw JM, Russell IT. Effect of clinical guidelines on medical practice: a systematic review of rigorous evaluations. *Lancet* 1993; 342: 1317-22.
9 Grimshaw JM, Russell IT. Achieving health gain through clinical guidelines. I. Developing scientifically valid guidelines. *Quality in Health Care* 1993; 2: 243-8.
10 Grimshaw JM, Russell IT. Achieving health gain through clinical guidelines. II. Ensuring that guidelines change medical practice. *Quality in Health Care* 1994; 3: 45-52.
11 Russell IT, Grimshaw J. The effectiveness of referral guidelines: a review of the methods and findings of published evaluations. In: Coulter A, Roland M, eds. *Referrals from general practice.* Oxford: Oxford University Press, 1992: 179-211.
12 Williams A. Purchasing outcomes: how should cost-effectiveness information influence clinical practice? In: *Outcomes into clinical practice.* London: BMJ Publishing Group, 1994: 99-107.
13 Grimshaw JM. Guidelines. *BMJ* 1994; 308: 1511.
14 Hayward RSA, Wilson MC, Tunis SR, Bass EB, Rubin HR, Haynes RB. More informative abstracts of articles describing clinical practice guidelines. *Ann Intern Med* 1993; 118: 731-7.
15 Smith R. Challenging doctors: an interview with England's chief medical officer. *BMJ* 1994; 308: 1221-4.
16 Lohr KN. Field MJ. Appendix B: a provisional instrument for assessing clinical practice guidelines. In: Institute of Medicine. *Guidelines for clinical practice: from development to use.* Washington, DC: National Academic Press. 1992: 346-410.
17 Grol R. Implementing guidelines in general practice care. *Quality in Health Care* 1992; 1: 184-91.
18 Mittman BS, Tonesk X, Jacobson PD. Implementing clinical practice guidelines: social influence strategies and practitioner behaviour change. *Qual Rev Bull* 1992; 18: 413-22.
19 Lomas J. *Teaching old (and not so old) docs new tricks: effective ways to implement research findings.* Toronto: McMaster University Centre for Health Economics and Policy Analysis, 1993. (Working paper 93-4)
20 Clinical Resource and Audit Group. *Clinical guidelines: a report by a working group set up by the Clinical Resource and Audit Group.* Edinburgh: Scottish Office, 1993.
21 McNichol M, Layton A, Morgan G. Team working: the key to implementing guidelines. *Quality in Health Care* 1993; 2: 215-6.
22 Williamson JA. Formulating priorities for quality assurance activity: description of a method and its application. *JAMA* 1978; 239: 631-7.
23 Fink A, Kosecoff J, Chassin M, Brook RH. Consensus methods: characteristics and guidelines for use. *Am J Public Health* 1984; 74: 979-83.
24 Irvine D, Donaldson L. Quality and standards in health care. In: Beck JS, Bouchier IAD, Russell IT, eds. *Quality assurance in medical care.* Edinburgh: Royal Society of Edinburgh, 1993: 1-30.

19 Reflections on key messages

DAVID J HUNTER

The title of the conference and this book is important – "Outcomes into Clinical Practice." The choice of the preposition "into" is significant since it is an attempt to capture the interface between the production of knowledge on the one hand and getting it into organisational and professional practice on the other. In this regard I think we may have underestimated the importance of both micropolitics and big politics in the discussion. As David Eddy, Professor of Health Policy and Management at the University of New Jersey, has put it, medicine is "a huge assumption." The rational scientific model which underpins most of what we think happens in medical practice is of limited utility. We need a different perspective in order to understand the dynamics of modern medicine.

Micropolitics

In relation to the micropolitical discussion, we need to give attention to the interplay of power between the key stakeholders, all of whom have been considered in the previous papers: professionals, policy makers and managers of policies, patients and consumers of health care, and researchers.

Research on effectiveness and outcomes research is not neutral in its impact – it can, and should, threaten the existing order and power balance, especially if we are serious about consumer

162

empowerment. Moreover, the research community is also empowered by the move towards taking outcomes seriously.

There is also an issue about equity if consumers are empowered: in particular, the collective ethos underpinning the NHS and its founding principles is in tension with the notion of the individual which is the essence of the consumerist movement. How the two are to be reconciled constitutes a major challenge to those who subscribe to the principle of equity. Moreover, even among users there is great heterogeneity. Users do not form a homogeneous group as far as health care is concerned.

Furthermore, there is the importance of managing change. This will not occur if imposed under a command and control model or if the bottom line is seen to be cost control. NHS Executive letter EL(93)115 is concerned with the issue of clinical effectiveness and guidelines, but its approach is inappropriate. It follows a top down model of management which is no longer seen to be relevant in a context in which there is supposed to be devolution to the frontline of care delivery. There is, therefore, an issue about from whose perspective the guidelines are seen to be effective or important. There are implications in all of this for professional education, training, and development. To date, medical schools have apparently been immune from the developments that have taken place in the health policy arena.

The importance of collaboration between purchasers and providers has been emphasised. Yet, does the competitive ethos being paraded in the NHS not work against the notion of collaboration? There is surely a contradiction here.

Meanwhile, competition is alive and well in the research community. I believe this is an unhealthy situation and one which militates against collaborative effort. There is a tension, for example, between the advocates of randomised controlled trials who believe that they constitute the gold standard of health services research on the one hand, and those who wish to understand and explain behaviour, whether on the part of professionals or consumers, on the other. We should not exclude the softer social sciences from making an important contribution to the debate about how to improve effectiveness and get outcomes into clinical practice. Studies have suggested that doctors do not act probabilistically but rather interpretatively. Discussions at this conference have highlighted the notion of "bothersomeness" in relation to how patients feel about their health. If the bothersomeness factor is to be captured in research it will require a more sociological approach to the concerns of patients than a mechanistic biomedical approach.

A further issue is the importance of outcomes for everybody rather than simply clinicians or managers. It is the business of the purchasing team, and indeed the providers, to take outcomes seriously. Relying on public health medicine alone to take the lead is insufficient.

Big politics

Finally, let me turn to the big politics issue. The post-1991 NHS is infused by a "can do, gung ho" culture. Ministers (and therefore managers) are impatient for results. Purchasers in particular are under considerable pressure to deliver health gain and yet time is not on their side. We are confronted with a paradoxical situation. Although welcome, the emphasis on effectiveness research and health outcomes is being articulated within a time frame that is quite unrealistic. This risks reducing the chances of achieving effective results. Ministers must acknowledge that seeing a research culture in the NHS will take longer than they, impatient for results, may be prepared to allow.

Getting outcomes into clinical practice will take time, as many of these chapters show. The process cannot be rushed if effective ownership among clinicians is to be secured. The infrastructure, mainly through the research and development initiative, is gradually being put into place. For this to produce results it will be important not to rush the developments that are now in hand. Arguably, purchasers and others are drowning in data and the issue is not so much one of identifying appropriate practice but of ensuring that the lessons are learnt in respect of future developments. Squaring this particular circle is perhaps the most urgent and difficult challenge that the outcomes movement faces. We should not ignore the fact that purchasers are on trial and have probably a year at most in which to deliver positive results. Should they fail to do so, I suspect we will see yet further change in the nature of the purchaser-provider separation in which the puchaser role gets radically redefined. Indeed, such a redefinition is already underway. The moves to merge DHAs and FHSAs, and to develop and extend general practice fundholding are not irrelevant in this debate.

Index